Biotechnology, weapons and humanity

Biotechnology, weapons and humanity

British Medical Association

TO BE
DISPOSED
BY
AUTHORITY

 harwood academic publishers

Australia • Canada • China • France • Germany • India
Japan• Luxembourg • Malaysia • The Netherlands • Russia
Singapore• Switzerland

Copyright © 1999 British Medical Association
Published by license under the Harwood Academic Publishers
imprint, part of the The Gordon and Breach Publishing Group.

Amsteldijk 166
1st Floor
1079 LH Amsterdam
The Netherlands

British Library Cataloguing in Publication Data
A catalogue record for this book is available from the British
Library.

ISBN 90-5702-460-8 (soft cover)

Cover photograph: TVF

Table of contents

Board of Science and Education

The report was prepared under the auspices of the Board of Science and Education of the British Medical Association. The members were:

Professor Sir Dillwyn Williams President, BMA
Professor B R Hopkinson Chairman of the Representative Body, BMA
Dr I G Bogle Chairman of Council, BMA
Dr W J Appleyard Treasurer, BMA
Sir William Asscher Chairman, Board of Science and Education
Dr P H Dangerfield Deputy Chairman, Board of Science and Education
Dr P Berry
Dr H W K Fell
Miss C E Fozzard
Dr S Hajioff
Dr V Leach
Dr N D L Olsen
Dr S J Richards
Dr S Somjee (from November 1998)
Dr P Steadman
Dr S Taylor
Dr D M B Ward

Acknowledgements

The Association is grateful for help provided by many individuals and organisations in the preparation of this document. We are extremely grateful for guidance provided by the Craft Committees, and Council members of the BMA. In particular we would like to thank Professor J W Almond and Dr Alastair Hay.

List of tables

List of figures

Acronyms

AHG	Ad Hoc Group
ARM	Annual Representative Meeting
BMA	British Medical Association
bp	base pair
BTWC	Biological and Toxin Weapons Convention
BW	Biological Weapons/Warfare
CB	Chemical and Biological
CBI	Confidential Business Information
CBW	Chemical and Biological Warfare
CFE	Conventional Forces in Europe
CIA	Central Intelligence Agency
COU	Concepts of use
CW	Chemical Warfare
CWC	Chemical Weapons Convention
DARPA	Defense Advanced Research Projects Agency (US)
DNA	Deoxyribonucleic acid
EAE	Ethnic-affiliation estimation
FFCD	Iraq's full, final and complete declaration
GMP	Good Manufacturing Practice
HGP	Human Genome Project
HIV	Human Immunodeficiency Virus
HUGO	Human Genome Organisation
ICC	International Criminal Court
ICRC	International Committee of the Red Cross
MRC	Medical Research Council
NATO	North Atlantic Treaty Organisation
NIH	National Institutes of Health
NPT	Nuclear Non-Proliferation Treaty

SIPRI	Stockholm International Peace Research Institute
SIrUS	Superfluous Injury or Unnecessary Suffering (project)
STRs	Short Tandem Repeats
TEM	Technical Evaluation Meeting
UK	United Kingdom
UN	United Nations
UNSCOM	United Nations Special Commission
US	United States
UV	Ultra violet
VEE	Venezuelan Equine Encephalomyelitis
VEREX	Ad Hoc Group of Governmental Experts to Identify and Examine Potential Verification Measures from a Scientific and Technical Standpoint
WHO	World Health Organisation
WMD	Weapons of mass destruction

Executive summary

- The world faces the prospect that the new revolution in biotechnology and medicine will find significant offensive military applications in the next century, just as the revolutions in chemistry and atomic physics did in the twentieth century.

- Biological weapons have been used sporadically in conflicts throughout history. They have been developed in line with scientific advances, making them increasingly potent agents. Since 1948 they have been categorised as weapons of mass destruction. Despite the 1925 Geneva Protocol and the 1975 Biological and Toxin Weapons Convention (BTWC) they are, in reality, poorly regulated and controlled.

- Prohibitions on the development and use of biological and toxin weapons have not been fully effective; intense and urgent efforts are needed to make the BTWC an effective instrument.

- Biological weapons may already be in the hands of a number of countries, and are also a realistic weapon for some terrorist groups. Control mechanisms must address not only the types of agents which might be used as weapons, and the protection against, and response to, their use, but also the ability of non-governmental groups to possess and use such weapons.

- Over the last few decades rapid advances in molecular biology have allowed the heritable material (DNA) of different organisms to be interchanged. The Human Genome Project and the Human Genetic Diversity Projects are allowing the identification of human genetic coding and differences in normal genetic material between different ethnic groups.

- During the review conferences on the BTWC, an increasing level of concern has been expressed by national governments over the potential use of genetic knowledge in the development of a new generation of biological and toxin weapons.

- Legitimate research into microbiological agents, relating both to the development of agents for use in, for example agriculture, or to improve the medical response to disease causing agents, may be difficult to distinguish from research with the malign purpose of producing more effective weapons.

- Scientists should recognise the pressures that can be brought to bear on them, and on their colleagues, to participate in the development of weapons.

- The recent history of conflict is predominantly of wars within states, often between different ethnic groups.

- Consideration of ethnic weapons have historically been based upon natural susceptibilities, or upon the absence of vaccination within a target group. Genetic engineering of biological agents, to make them more potent, has been carried out covertly for some years, but not as an overt step to produce more effective weapons. In genetic terms there are more similarities between different people and peoples than there are differences. But the differences exist, and may singly or in combination distinguish the members of one social group (an "ethnic" group) from another.

- Research into the development of specific treatments for many medical conditions (both genetic and acquired) using genetic knowledge and genetic techniques, is currently consuming a significant proportion of the pharmacological research budget internationally. This research considers essentially the same molecular techniques as would weapons development.

- There are massive imbalances between states in the availability and sophistication of weapons, both conventional and nuclear. This is no reason for delaying further the establishment of effective measures to control the proliferation of biological weapons.

- Processes to enhance and strengthen the existing Biological and Toxin Weapons Convention are essential to prevent the further spread of the current generation of biological weapons. Effective monitoring and verification procedures would also be powerful controls against the development of genetically targeted biological weapons.

- Modern biotechnology and medicine have essential roles in improving the quality of life for people in the developed and developing world; molecular medicine has much to offer people throughout the world. Procedures to monitor against the abuse/malign use of this knowledge and technology may also contribute significantly to the development of effective disease surveillance programmes.

- 'Recipes' for developing biological agents are freely available on the Internet. As genetic manipulation becomes a standard laboratory technique this information is also likely to be widely available. The window of opportunity for developing effective controls is thus fairly narrow.

- The medical profession has played a significant part in the development of International Humanitarian Law, especially through the International Committee of the Red Cross (ICRC). The work of doctors with the ICRC on the SIrUS project offers real hope of an extension of this area of law to reduce the suffering which might be caused by new weapons technology.

- Realistically doctors should accept that even with effective international legal instruments, some weapons development with molecular biological knowledge will go ahead. Doctors must therefore be prepared to recognise and respond to the use of such weapons, and to advise governments on plans and policies to minimise their effect.

- Urgent action is essential to ensure that the BTWC is strengthened, and to reinforce the central concept that biological weapons, whether simple or complex in design and production, are wholly unacceptable.

• The physician's role is the prevention and treatment of disease. The deliberate use of disease or chemical toxins is directly contrary to the medical profession's whole ethos and rationale. Such misuse must be stigmatised so that it is completely rejected by civilised society.

• There is a need for Government action at a national and international level to complete effective, verifiable and enforceable agreements and countermeasures before the proliferation and development of new biological weapons makes this almost impossible. Doctors and scientists have an important role to play in campaigning for, and enforcing, adequate preventive measures. The Board of Science and Education's recommendations for achieving these goals can be found in Chapter 7.

CHAPTER 1

Introduction

British Medical Association and the Board of Science and Education

The British Medical Association (BMA) is the professional organisation representing all doctors in the UK. The BMA Board of Science and Education undertakes research studies on behalf of the BMA and has facilitated debate on key public health and professional issues.

Doctors are professionally committed to the avoidance of human injury and disease, but will be called upon to deal with the human consequences of weapons used in wars and terrorist attacks. This report considers the role of doctors as well as scientists, governments and international agencies, in limiting and managing the effects of weapons use and limiting the use of weapons which cause unacceptable damage/injuries to individuals and to populations.

In particular, we are concerned that the emerging sciences of genetic engineering and biotechnology may be developed for malign purposes. The social and ethical safeguards which may prevent the escalation of conflict and weapons development therefore need to be discussed urgently. This report hopes to stimulate debate and raise civic awareness of the potential abuse of biotechnology and the important steps that we can take to minimise the risk of the development of biological weapons.

Weapons, ethics and the BMA

The Board of Science and Education has published policy reports on *The Medical Effects of Nuclear War*[1] (1983), *Nuclear Attack: Ethics and Casualty Selection*[2] (1988) and *The Medical Implications of Chemical and Biological Warfare*[3] (1987). These reports took an apolitical stance on weapons, but stated quite clearly the medical consequences of their use. More recently, the BMA has taken an active part in the campaign to ban anti-personnel landmines. As doctors within the military and humanitarian aid agencies began to consider the landmines case, and following the recent success of achieving an agreement to ban the use of blinding laser weapons, surgeons at the International Committee of the Red Cross (ICRC) began to draw together a panel of experts to prepare objective medical criteria by which the effects of individual weapons could be assessed. Their remit was to consider weapons which cause Superfluous Injury or Unnecessary Suffering (SIrUS project). The SIrUS group received a number of papers addressing current weapons and weapons research. It was apparent that almost all scientific advances have been historically considered for their weapons potential and that the medical knowledge obtained from the Human Genome Project could be used for malign purposes.

The work of the SIrUS group has now been published[4] and medical organisations and associations invited to endorse its findings. In July 1998, the Ministry of Defence of the United Kingdom announced that the moratorium on the use of anti-personnel landmines had become a total ban. Genetic knowledge and weapons are not a substantive part of the final report from the SIrUS project, although it has generated interest in the role doctors could have in preventing the spread of a new generation of weapons which cause superfluous injury or unnecessary suffering. The BMA is particularly concerned about knowledge that might lead to the development of weapons which may target specific ethnic or racial groups, in view of the nature of the majority of current and recent conflicts.

Biological weapons

We now know that soon after the 'Golden Age' of microbiology, efforts were made to use anthrax as a biological weapon (see Appendix 1) during the First World War.[5] The 1925 Geneva Protocol, which was negotiated in the decade following that war, prohibited the first use of biological weapons, but not their development. Biological weapons have been the subject of large-scale scientific research throughout the last 70 years. There is considerable evidence that some countries are still undertaking research into more effective weapons and delivery systems.

Recent advances in genetic research raise the spectre of targeted versions of biological weapons. Biological weapons have not been used on more of the world's battlefields, in part, because they generally affect all who breathe them or are otherwise exposed in their delivery mechanism. A system of specific targeting would make these weapons more usable in military terms.

The international law and conventions surrounding research on genetic weapons, as well as their use, is that which controls biological weapons generally. It therefore holds that strengths and weaknesses of those systems of control will apply equally for genetic weapons. We have therefore decided to examine the strengths and weaknesses of the Biological and Toxin Weapons Convention (BTWC) as an integral part of this report.

The BTWC of 1972, whilst prohibiting the development, production, stockpiling or acquisition of biological weapons, had no effective means of verification.[6] Offensive biological weapons programmes were therefore left unregulated by international arms control agreements (see Appendix 2) at precisely the time when the revolution in modern biotechnology began. Given the revelations about such programmes in Iraq[7] and the former Soviet Union,[8] it is not surprising that the 1996 Montreux Symposium of the International Committee of the Red Cross, on "The Medical Profession and the Effects of Weapons", had a working group where the discussion of future weapons:[9]

3

"*...concentrated particularly on biotechnology and the potential use of genetic research, which seems to be very much in the weapons threshold category.*"

The Symposium concluded that:

"*...weapons of the future, especially those developed on the basis of knowledge of the human genome and of genetic engineering, should be given serious consideration...*"

Following the Montreux Symposium, and the expression of similar concerns at the 48th World Medical Association General Assembly in South Africa in October 1996,[10] the British Medical Association decided to commission a report to investigate this topic in more detail, with a view to making recommendations on how the development and possible use of biological weapons might be better prevented — particularly by actions that might be undertaken by the medical profession. Whilst a number of aspects of international law impinge on the regulation of biological warfare,[11] it is clear that the major issue at the present time is whether the BTWC can be strengthened by addition of the Verification Protocol presently under negotiation by the States Parties. Thus the analysis and recommendations here are centred on the evolution of the BTWC regulatory regime.

However, legislation alone is not enough to control the use of weapons. Many weapons are in the control of governments, but vast numbers are controlled by guerilla forces, criminals and terrorists. The only way to prevent the abuse of a weapon is to prevent its production, manufacture and sale, and closely monitor the work of scientists to ensure that their work is not used for malign purposes.

Recent advances in genetics

The Human Genome Project is mapping the genes which code for human structure and function. The Human Genetic Diversity

Project describes those normal variants which exist in different populations. This second project is designed to provide information on a number of the most endangered human population groups, but related work demonstrates the population subgroups within many different countries.

The similarities between different populations are generally more significant than the differences, but the differences are significant, and by combining a series of factors the projects will deliver information allowing selective identification and potential targeting of disparate ethnic and familial groups. The research which develops specific therapeutic agents is scientifically (but not ethically) indistinguishable from research to develop a lethal or disabling agent targeted at specific clusters of genes or alleles.

It follows that any mechanism for preventing the development of such agents must also monitor developments in laboratories carrying out medical and therapeutic research. This must also include monitoring and mentoring by peer groups to ensure that researchers are not persuaded or coerced into carrying out weapons research. Doctors and scientists must understand the regulation and control systems in order to prohibit the abuse of their scientific discoveries.

Structure and scope of report

The aim of the report is to consider new developments in biotechnology, especially human genetics, which could be incorporated into the available weaponry of nation states and terrorist organisations. In particular, the report considers whether weapons could be based on genetic knowledge and if so, how legislation and other measures could prevent such a malign use of scientific knowledge.

This chapter sets out the aims and objectives of the report within the context of concern shown by the medical profession at the 48th WMA meeting held in South Africa in 1996. Chapter 2 provides a history of offensive biological weapons programmes and of international arms control efforts in the twentieth century to prohibit such programmes. Chapter 3 then outlines the major features of the modern biotechnology revolution and why this has caused such concerns about the possible development of new biological weapons. As an example of these concerns, the possible development of 'ethnic' weapons based on advances in our understanding of human genetics and targeted at specific racial/ethnic groups is examined in Chapter 4. In Chapter 5 the currently available mechanisms of control of offensive biological weapons programmes are described, and in Chapter 6 suggestions for further measures to help deter states and organisations from developing such weapons are reviewed. Chapter 7 presents recommendations for action and further research by the scientific and medical community, both nationally and also on an international basis.

As will become apparent, biological weapons come in many forms and can be used in many different ways. However, the main cause for concern is that these weapons, which are basically unregulated and rather easy to develop, could proliferate in areas of regional instability, or enter the available weaponry of terrorists. Such proliferation should be viewed in the context that since 1948 the United Nations have considered biological weapons as weapons of mass destruction, ie in the same category as nuclear weapons.[12]

This report discusses the relationship between medicine, biotechnology and humanity. It considers the development of weapons which may become a major threat to the existence of *Homo sapiens*, and a development of biotechnology which perverts the humanitarian nature of biomedical science. It is all the more frightening that medical professionals may contribute, willingly or unwittingly, to the development of new, potent weapons. This potential for malign use of biomedical knowledge also places responsibility on doctors and scientists to protect the integrity of their work.

Genetic engineering can be of great benefit to medical science and humanity, but can also be used for harm. Genetic information is already being used to improve elements of biological weapons —

such as increased antibiotic resistance — and it is likely that this trend will accelerate as the knowledge and understanding of its applications become more widely known, unless effective control systems can be agreed. The pattern of scientific development is such that developing effective control systems within the next five to ten years will be crucial to future world security.

CHAPTER 2

The history of biological warfare

As the threat of biological warfare has become a growing concern there have been greater efforts made to understand the nature of this form of warfare by a fuller investigation of its history. Rather than being an occasional and ineffective method of warfare, the history of biological warfare points to it being pervasive, and offering extensive future possibilities. Poupard and Miller,[1] whilst accepting that it is often difficult to obtain definitive proof of the use of biological warfare prior to 1900 from the historical record, suggest that it is possible to see the evolution of biological warfare over time in six historical periods. It is convenient to use this division in the following brief overview of the history of biological warfare. An attempt is then made to construct a typology of potential uses of biological and toxin weapons. It should be noted however that description of the various biological warfare programmes will, for simplicity, concentrate on the offensive aspect, that is, on efforts to develop weapons. A full description would require detailed analysis of efforts to develop defence against biological weapons — detection, protection etc — but that is beyond the remit of the present study.

From 300 BC to 1763

In developing a proper concept of biological warfare, it is important that practice in antiquity is taken into account. The Greeks, Romans and Persians polluted the water supplies of their enemies with animal corpses. This was a calculated means of denying the essential water needed by all armies. There is also considerable evidence of the use of catapults, during the medieval period, to hurl diseased bodies into besieged cities in order to spread infection and force surrender.

1763 to 1925

A significant change took place in 1763, when there is documented use of a specific disease — smallpox — by the British against North American Indians. Wheelis, who uses a stringent set of criteria in assessing the occurrence of biological warfare in the historical record, accepts this example as proven.[2] The method used was the deliberate transfer of infected blankets to the Indians. The background to this incident, and other possible examples of the same kind, was the devastating impact of European diseases — particularly smallpox — on the native North American Indian populations. The European settlement of North America was thus a *re*settlement following, as contemporary European accounts record, widespread deaths amongst the original populations from natural infection. In short, the infected blankets incident is an example of attempted genocide/ethnic cleansing, using biological weapons. As the British Commander-in-Chief[3] expressed it, in a letter of 1763 to his regional commander for the Pennsylvania frontier, "[Y]ou will do well to try to inoculate the Indians by means of blankets, as well as to try every other method that can serve to extirpate this execrable race".

Despite such examples, van Courtland Moon, in an extended historical review of legal restraints,[4] has argued that there has long been a strong prohibition against the use of biological weapons because of their relationship to chemical weapons and the general abhorrence of the use of poison. This prohibition had become a principal of customary international law by the end of the classical Greek and Roman period and, following better definition of the prohibition from the seventeenth century, it was beginning to become codified in the latter half of the nineteenth century. Thus Article 70 of the Lieber code,[5] drafted to regulate warfare during the US Civil War, states that:

> *"The use of poison in any manner, be it to poison wells, or food, or arms, is wholly excluded from modern warfare. He that uses it puts himself out of the pale of law and usages of war."*

This code influenced thinking subsequently in Europe, and was reflected in the International Declaration concerning the Laws and Customs of War signed in Brussels in 1874 which, although never ratified, fed directly into the First and Second International Peace Conferences in The Hague in 1899 and 1907 respectively. Boserup, in the 1970s Stockholm International Peace Research Institute (SIPRI) study of "CBW [Chemical and Biological Warfare] and the Law of War", pointed out that the records of the Brussels Conference demonstrated that the reference to poison and poison weapons clearly included the spreading of disease.[6]

The development of the science of microbiology in the late nineteenth century had considerably extended the potential scope of biological warfare, as the specific agents and mechanisms of disease and disease prevention became better known.[7,8] Thus German use of biological warfare in the First World War was directed at a number of countries with the aim of sabotaging valuable allied horse stocks and also grain shipments, an example of anti-animal and anti-plant biological warfare (Table 2.1).

Despite most of the German records having been destroyed or lost there is no doubt that biological sabotage was directed by the General Staff.[10] It must also have been preceded by a dedicated research and development programme devoted to determining how the agents could be transported and used effectively.

11

Table 2.1: German offensive anti-animal and anti-plant biological warfare in the First World War*

Date	Place	Target	Agents
1915-16	Eastern seaboard of US	Horse shipments to Europe	Anthrax and glanders
1915-16	Romania	Horses and livestock	Anthrax and glanders
1916	Norway	Reindeer draft animals	Anthrax
1917	Western Front	Horses	Anthrax
1917-18	Argentina	Horse shipments to Europe	Anthrax and glanders
		Stored grain	Fungus

*From[9]

We know most about the German biological campaign against the United States because it was part of a much larger general sabotage campaign that was later the subject of legal proceedings. The adjudication of the US claims for losses in the sabotage campaign was not finally resolved until just before the Second World War, but the records allow an account to be given of the biological aspect of the overall sabotage campaign. Anthrax and glanders agents (an infectious disease of horses) were cultured from seed stocks by the principal German operative in the US, packaged and then distributed to local personnel, who jabbed the horses with infected needles. The campaign in South America against both animal and grain shipments was again, of course, at extremely long range and involved shipments of biological agents in part by U-boat. It is worth noting that British naval intelligence was following this operation through the decoding of German wireless telegraph transmissions and made attempts to interfere with its progress. The less well known German campaign in Romania was somewhat easier to carry out because material could be shipped overland through friendly countries.

Most of the documentation on the French biological warfare programme before the Second World War was destroyed in 1940 to prevent it falling into German hands. The account we currently have is therefore incomplete.[11] It is known, however, that at a meeting of a Bacteriological Commission in the War Ministry in December 1923, Veterinary Inspector Vallée stated:

> *"...that he had had the opportunity during the Great War to prepare a virus that was inoffensive to man but easily inoculable in the horse, and which caused an infectious anaemia. This virus had been used against the enemy cavalry..."*

The word virus was not being used by Vallée in the modern sense, and the agent was probably glanders.[12] The Germans certainly believed that they were attacked by the French with biological weapons.

Whatever the nature of French biological warfare during the First World War, there is no doubt that serious attention was paid to the subject immediately afterwards. Three phases of research can be detected between the wars: 1921-26; 1927-34; and 1935-40. The first and third phases of interest and activity were triggered by French perceptions of German interest in biological warfare, whilst the second phase, of low levels of activity, was triggered by French concern to be seen to be living up to the obligations embodied in the 1925 Geneva Protocol. The French work, up to 1927, seems to have foreshadowed much of what was to follow in later programmes. There was clearly careful selection of suitable agents, consideration of the most efficient means of military use and then effective weaponisation. Weaponisation was a significant step because military use requires a means of delivering large amounts of agent to a target. Given the fragility of microorganisms, developing an effective weapon to deliver agents was a complex task.

1925 to 1940

Following the widespread employment of deadly chemical weapons during the First World War, it is not surprising that strenuous efforts were made when the war ended, to prevent them ever being used again.[13] Eventually, the 1925 Geneva Protocol (Table 2.2) was agreed.

Table 2.2: The 1925 Geneva Protocol*

Protocol for the Prohibition of the Use in War of Asphyxiating, Poisonous or other Gases, and of Bacteriological Methods of Warfare. Signed at Geneva on 19 June 1925

The Undersigned Plenipotentiaries, in the name of their respective Governments,

Whereas the use in war of asphyxiating, poisonous or other gases, and of all analogous liquids, materials or devices, has been justly condemned by the general opinion of the civilized world; and

Whereas the prohibition of such use has been declared in Treaties to which the majority of the Powers of the world are Parties; and

To the end that this prohibition shall be universally accepted as a part of International Law, binding alike the conscience and the practice of nations;

Declare:

That the High Contracting Parties, so far as they are not already Parties to Treaties prohibiting such use, accept this prohibition, agree to extend this prohibition to the use of bacteriological methods of warfare and agree to be bound as between themselves according to the terms of this declaration...

*From[14]

The Protocol is, in effect, a no-first-use agreement between states which has now essentially become a part of customary international law. During the drafting of the Protocol the Polish delegate pointed out the omission of bacteriological warfare. This, he argued, had been included in the discussions and was important because the agents were simpler and cheaper to produce than chemicals and could have significant long-term effects. This argument was accepted and led to the inclusion of the reference to "bacteriological methods of warfare" in the prohibition. This is an extremely general ban that clearly includes anti-plant and anti-animal warfare, as well as attacks on human beings. The term 'bacteriological' is now of course, taken to cover all biological agents.[15] The Protocol has a number of weaknesses; in particular, it did not prevent biological warfare being researched or preparations being made for its use — at least in retaliation. Thus the offensive biological research and development carried out by states in the middle years of this century was not banned by the 1925 Protocol.

Many military establishments took the possibility of biological warfare very seriously prior to the Second World War. For example, in Hungary there was a secret biological warfare programme running from 1936 to 1944 which has recently been described.[16] The programme involved a central institute in Budapest with eight microbiological and one chemical laboratory. The Hungarian programme shows consideration of the most efficient means of military use and careful agent selection, as in the earlier first phase of the French programme.

In attempting to understand the potential dangers we face, it is necessary to confront the inhumanity of Japanese offensive biological warfare. As Colonel Mobley USAR has pointed out, the Geneva Protocol had the unintended effect of suggesting to a Japanese officer, Ishii Shiro, that if use of biological weapons was banned in an international agreement they must be effective.[17] Ishii Shiro and his colleagues then launched "perhaps the most gruesome series of BW experiments in history" which involved the deliberate infection and certain death of large numbers of human captives within occupied China. When the Soviet Union put a number of the lesser perpetrators on trial after the war, the facts were not generally accepted in the West. Much information has now become available and it is clear that the United States negotiated with Ishii Shiro and the others primarily in charge to grant them immunity from prosecution in exchange for the knowledge they had gained. The US position, according to Sheldon Harris, who has provided the most recent English language description,[18] was encapsulated in a 1947 dispatch which stated:

> *"Evidence gathered in this investigation has greatly supplemented and amplified previous aspects of this field....Information has accrued with respect to human susceptibility to those diseases as indicated by specific doses of bacteria. Such information could not be obtained in our own laboratories because of the scruples attached to human experimentation..."*

One of the ironies of this covert deal, according to Harris, is that the information proved to be of limited value to the Americans as the major US offensive biological warfare programme developed after the war. There is no doubt, however, that the Japanese programme which began in the early 1930s was on a massive scale and involved large numbers of scientists and doctors. As the scientists and doctors involved were rotated periodically, thousands must have been involved in human experimentation and many of these were civilians who joined the units voluntarily.[19] Effects of an enormous range of pathogens and toxins on humans, animals and plants were studied by Ishii Shiro and his collaborators, and laboratory testing involved an unknown number, probably many thousands, of human victims. More of those who carried out the dreadful experimentation have come forward recently to record their experiences and regrets, and to try to give some explanation for their behaviour.[20]

Given the scale of this programme, it is not surprising that it led to extensive efforts at weaponisation of agents,[21] and to attempts to *use* biological weapons in the field. Allegations of such use in China during the Second World War were certainly known about at high levels in the Western Alliance[22] and have subsequently been confirmed.[23,24,25] The field testing of biological warfare in a variety of different ways was attempted. In the period 1939-1942, at least twelve biological warfare field tests were carried out.[26] Many of these trials were as sabotage (or terrorism) directed against the civilian Chinese population, but efforts were also made to develop means of effective, large-scale, military use of biological weapons through bombing.

The British view at the end of the war, in regard to Japanese weaponisation, was that the Japanese had expended considerable effort in attempting to produce an effective weapon.[27] However, the operational problems in the effective use of these bombs were never solved. According to the British report, it is significant that:

> *"...the authorities...disregarded any possible need for accumulation of quantitative data in cloud chambers preliminary to setting up field trials. (Indeed, such chamber studies were never attempted)..."*

Thus the data available to later offensive biological warfare programmes, from the developing science of aerobiology, was not available to the Japanese.

1940 to 1969

In contrast to Japan, the investigations carried out by the Western allies after the Second World War revealed that during the inter-war years Germany had not given any serious consideration to the possible use of biological weapons.[28] Moreover, during the Second World War, German efforts in the field of biological warfare were limited, badly co-ordinated and only activated in response to information received about Allied activities, for example about French work after the fall of France in 1940, and when full documentation of French work was discovered in 1942. Specific instructions were issued from the highest levels restricting preparations *solely* to defence against possible attack. Nevertheless, some offensive work was carried out, particularly on anti-plant agents, by the agricultural section of the BW organisation, either because directives were misunderstood or ignored, or in order to make more effective defensive preparations.

Despite the lack of German work on biological warfare in the 1930s, intelligence reports about German interest in the subject led to increasing concern in Britain and to the establishment in

1936 of a Biological Warfare Sub-Committee of the Committee of Imperial Defence. High-level concern was maintained for many years, particularly through the influence of the Secretary of the Committee of Imperial Defence, Lord Hankey.[29] Hankey himself wrote a key paper[30] after the outbreak of war, "identifying the need for studies on BW to leave the realm of hypothesis and enter that of practical experiment". Dr Paul Fildes, who had previously worked at the Middlesex Hospital's Institute of Pathology,[31] was appointed to lead the effort. The British view was that they needed a biological weapon in order to be able to retaliate in kind, if threatened. This capability was achieved first by the production of an anti-animal weapon against German livestock. The plan was to drop anthrax-infected cattle cakes across agricultural land devoted to grazing, in sufficient numbers to achieve effective concentrations over a given period. Tests had shown that cattle would locate the cattle cakes and that, in the process of eating the cakes, they would become infected by inhalation of the anthrax spores. By April 1943 five million infected cattle cakes were stored, ready for use. Had they been used, they would have been dropped from bombers over Germany. However, this was not the main line of future biological warfare opened up by Fildes.

Britain, of course, had extensive experience of the use of chemical weapons from the First World War and Fildes spent a good deal of time consulting experts on the use of these weapons, in an effort to find the most effective military use of biological weapons. By November 1940:[32]

> *"...Fildes had determined that the most effective way would be to disseminate an aerosol of lung-retention size particles from a liquid suspension of bacteria in a bursting munition such as a bomb, delivered so that effective concentrations would be inhaled by anyone in the target area..."*

Fildes concentrated work on anthrax and to a lesser extent on botulinum toxin, and this approach defined the main method of anti-human biological warfare through the rest of the century. In contrast to the Japanese approach to the problem of weaponisation, here it was determined that a rigorous quantitative experimental approach was needed. To this end, methods for the large-scale production of bacteria, controlled exposure of experimental animals to bacterial aerosols and field trials were rapidly developed.

The British programme progressed quickly and concentrated on the development of an anthrax (N-bomb) weapon for use against people. In 1942 and 1943 the British Government tested anthrax bombs on Gruinard Island off the northwest coast of Scotland. Gruinard was only returned to civilian use in 1990 — 47 years after the test. Field trials in 1942 demonstrated that "the weapon appeared to be more potent than any CW agent or munition of like size yet examined".[33] The superior effectiveness of biological weapons over chemical weapons has been repeatedly demonstrated and clearly places biological weapons in a category with nuclear weapons in terms of potential lethality.[34]

By this time, however, the three-way collaboration between the US, Canada and Britain was underway and in May 1943 Fildes had all of the British data transferred to the US and Canada.[35] The requirement for an effective means of retaliation against the perceived probability of German use of biological weapons[36] was to be met by a joint project in which the US would undertake production and Canada large-scale field testing. The project was not completed by the end of the war, but the thinking behind the project can be gathered from a 1945 note[37] by the Joint Secretaries of the Joint Technical Warfare Committee of the UK Chiefs of Staff Committee (Table 2.3).

British concern about biological warfare remained high after the war with, even in that time of severe financial restraint, massive expenditure on a new state-of-the-art microbiology building at Porton Down and extensive field trials at sea off the UK and off the Bahamas. The British offensive biological warfare programme ended in the late 1950s,[38] but by that time the US programme dwarfed the British efforts.

The history of the US programme and its results are well known, in large part because of the comparative openness of the US political system.[40] Important internal histories[41] and position

Table 2.3: British view of the anthrax (N-bomb) project in late 1945*

1. The position of BW research and development at the moment is as follows: One weapon (N) has been developed and has reached the initial stages of production...

2. N. is an A/C 500-lb cluster bomb containing 106 special bombs charged [with] anthrax spores. It is designed for strategic bombing as a reprisal. Detailed assessments have been considered ...

   (i) In general it has been thought that if 6 major German cities were attacked simultaneously by 2000 Lincolns armed with this weapon, 50% of the inhabitants who were exposed to the cloud of anthrax without respirators might be killed by inhalation, while many more might die through subsequent contamination of the skin...

   There is no danger of endemic spread.

   (ii) The terrain will be contaminated for years, and danger from skin infection should be great enough to enforce evacuation...

*From[39]

papers,[42] as well as technical documents,[43] have been available to scholars for many years. Thus although a great deal of historical research undoubtedly remains to be done,[44] the main outlines of the programme and its results are known. According to the standard US Army account,[45] the programme went through a series of phases following its initiation during the Second World War (Table 2.4).

The phases of activity were clearly linked to the ongoing state of the Cold War with the Soviet Union and the major wars in which the US was engaged. Whilst the US did not sign the Geneva Protocol until the offensive programme was over, it had made its position clear — at least in regard to chemical weapons only being available for retaliation — during the Second World War. A substantive change of policy was made in the mid-1950s. As the US Army account puts it:[47]

> *"...In 1956, a revised BW/CW policy was formulated to the effect that the US would be prepared to use BW or CW in a general war to enhance military effectiveness..."*

Table 2.4: The phases of the US offensive biological warfare programme*

Dates	Activity
1946-49	Research and planning years after World War II
1950-53	Expansion of the BW program during the Korean War
1954-58	Cold War years - reorganisation of weapons and defense programs
1959-62	Limited war period - expanded research, development, testing and operational readiness
1963-68	Adaptation of the BW program to counter insurgencies - the Vietnam War years
1969-73	Disarmament and phase down

*From[46]

In short, use of biological weapons would not be restricted to the deterrence of use by the threat of retaliation.

It was clearly understood in the early years of the programme that much could be gained from well-organised research and development. A report by the Ad Hoc Committee on Biological Warfare noted in 1949 that biological warfare was at a primitive stage and many improvements could be made.[48] Such improvements were delivered, the data suggesting an increase in efficiency of four orders of magnitude between 1940 and 1965.[49] It is against that background of increasing efficiency of production, storage, and distribution from munitions[50] that a number of anti-personnel and anti-plant agents were produced in large quantities. The official account summarises as follows:[51]

> *"...Between 1954 and 1967 the facility [Pine Bluff Arsenal] produced the following biological agents and toxins:* Brucella suis, Pasturella tularensis, *Q fever rickettsia, Venezuelan Equine Encephalomyelitis [VEE],* Bacillus anthracis, *botulinum toxin and staphylococcal enterotoxin. Bulk agents and antipersonnel munitions filled*

> with these various agents and toxins were produced and
> stored..."

In addition:

> "...Three anticrop biological agents were produced between
> 1951 and 1969. These included both stem rust of wheat
> and rye, and rice blast..."

The interest in incapacitating biological weapons (such as Q
fever and VEE virus) and in (chemical) toxins derived from micro-
organisms should be noted. Indeed, the overall results of the US
programme appear to support the view that "BW offers an almost
endless variety of ways to wage war".[52]

1969 to 1990

Notwithstanding the extensive American programme, President
Nixon decided to renounce unilaterally both biological and toxin
weapons, and the international community moved to agree the
Biological and Toxin Weapons Convention (BTWC), which
entered into force in 1975. In this Convention each State Party
undertakes:

> "...never in any circumstances to develop, produce, stockpile
> or otherwise acquire or retain:
>
> 1. Microbial or other biological agents, or toxins whatever
>   their origin or method of production, of types and in
>   quantities that have no justification for prophylactic,
>   protective or other peaceful purposes..."

The problem is that the Convention included no means of
verifying that the parties were living up to the obligations they had
undertaken.[53] In fact, evidence suggests that the Soviet Union
intensified their biological weapons programme after signing the
BTWC. The lack of verification measures — and the opportunity

this presents to evade the rules of the Convention — has caused increasing concern and resulted in current efforts to develop a Verification Protocol (see Chapter 5).

It has been argued that the United States renounced biological weapons because they were militarily insignificant, given the large scale development of nuclear weapons by the major powers. On this argument, the way was therefore open for negotiated disarmament: elimination of these potential means of mass destruction. The British expert Gradon Carter has strongly opposed such a suggestion, arguing instead that:[54]

> "...*The abandonment of BW arose from political considerations....The utility of BW had been demonstrated by all possible means, short of use in war, and the established feasibility could clearly not become disestablished with time...*"

Carter was particularly scathing about the argument that biological weapons were not useful because they caused epidemics. This, he pointed out, would only be a risk if particular agents were deliberately chosen (see Table 2.3 for the early British military view on anthrax, for example). It *could* be argued that there was every reason for the US to abandon the biological warfare programme because it was demonstrating to poorer, less technologically developed states, which would not be able to produce nuclear weapons, how to obtain weapons of mass destruction.

The US programme continued in a 'defence only' mode. When biological weapons are a possible threat, defensive research and development in relation to detection, protection, identification and prophylaxis are, of course, necessary and are clearly allowed by the BTWC. The benefits of such research have been well argued,[55] but they have also been questioned because of the potential difficulty of distinguishing defensive from offensive research.[56] The danger is that the objectives of defensive research could be misunderstood and thus provoke another state into a mistaken retaliatory offensive programme in response.

There can be no doubt that anyone who wished to know the basic facts about the effects of biological weapons could consult the comprehensive UN[57] and WHO[58] documents produced in the run-up to the negotiation of the BTWC. In order to be useful as biological weapons agents, the organisms would be required to have certain characteristics, for example high infectivity and high rates of survival in the environment (Table 2.5).

Table 2.5: Some militarily-desirable characteristics of biological weapons*

1. An agent should produce a known effect consistently.

2. The dose needed to produce the effect should be low.

3. There should be a short and predictable incubation period.

4. The target population should have little or no immunity.

5. Treatment for the disease should not be easily available to the target population.

6. The user should have means to protect troops and civilians.

7. It should be possible to easily mass produce the agent.

8. It should be possible to disseminate the agent efficiently.

9. The agent should be stable in storage and in munitions.

*From[59]

As a recent US Army study of proliferation pointed out, there are many agents (see also Appendix 3) with the required characteristics:[60]

> "...Of the approximately 160 known disease-causing species that directly or indirectly affect man, about 30 have been discussed in the open literature as having BW potential..."

It is not difficult to see why, in view of such abundant possibilities, military establishments in conflict-prone regions of the world should have maintained an interest in biological weapons. The US Congress Office of Technology Assessment[61] suggested in 1993 that eight countries in the Middle East and East Asia were generally considered to have undeclared offensive biological weapons programmes. Whilst the exact meaning of the accusations are frequently not clear, there has obviously been increasing official concern over proliferation of what is potentially a weapon of mass destruction (Table 2.6). Clearly, if 100 kg of anthrax spores spread effectively over a city in the right conditions might kill 1 to 3 million people, proliferation of such weapons must be of great concern.

Table 2.6: The effects of attacks with weapons of mass destruction*

Weapon system	Effect (number of deaths)
i) 1.0 Mt hydrogen bomb	570,000-1,900,000
ii) 1,000 kg Sarin nerve gas (line source with agent drifting on wind over target)	
(a) Clear, sunny day, light breeze	300-700
(b) Overcast day or night, moderate wind	400-800
(c) Clear, calm night	3,000-8,000
iii) 100 kg anthrax spores (line source with agent drifting on wind over target)	
(a) Clear, sunny day, light breeze	130,000-460,000
(b) Overcast day or night, moderate wind	420,000-1,400,000
(c) Clear, calm night	1,000,000-3,000,000

*From[62]

In recent years official statements relating to specific threats have become much more direct. For example, in a written answer to Congress in 1996, the Central Intelligence Agency (CIA) stated that Iran has had a biological warfare programme since 1980.[63] However, the most important indicator we have of the proliferation of biological weapons is the Iraqi programme uncovered by the United Nations Special Commission (UNSCOM) inspectors following the 1991 Gulf War. According to the most detailed UNSCOM report yet available on the nature of this programme:[64]

> *"Iraq's biological weapons programme as described to the Commission embraced a comprehensive range of agents and munitions. Agents under Iraq's biological weapons programme included lethal agents, eg anthrax, botulinum toxin and ricin, and incapacitating agents, eg aflatoxin, mycotoxins, haemorrhagic conjunctivitis virus and rotavirus. The scope of biological warfare agents worked on by Iraq encompassed both anti-personnel and anti-plant weapons..."*

The report continued:

> *"...The programme covered a whole variety of biological weapons delivery means, from tactical weapons (eg 122 mm rockets and artillery shells), to strategic weapons (eg aerial bombs and Al Hussein warheads filled with anthrax, botulinum toxin and aflatoxin) and 'economic' weapons, eg wheat cover smut..."*

Whilst later information suggests that Iraq's weapon systems were relatively crude and ineffective in 1991, it also suggests that they would not have taken long to solve the remaining problems of producing and disseminating agent in dry form from efficient dispensers.[65] Significantly, the UNSCOM report noted that:

> *"...authority to launch biological...warheads was pre-delegated in the event that Baghdad was hit by nuclear weapons during the Gulf war. This pre-delegation does not exclude the alternative use of such capability and therefore does not constitute proof of only intentions concerning second use..."*

Biological weapons, in short, may have been considered by the Iraqis as possible adjuncts to regular military operations but more probably as last-ditch deterrents against nuclear forces. Still in 1998, in the absence of a proper account of Iraq's biological weapons programme, there remains intense speculation over the agents developed and the operational planning for the use of these weapons.[66]

From the evidence available at present it is probably best to categorise Iraq's programme with the other large-scale state programmes of the middle years of the century. If we consider the sabotage attempts during the First World War as *first generation* biological warfare, then the programmes initiated in the 1920s and culminating in the massive US offensive biological programme, might be considered as *second generation*. These programmes, which concluded before 1970, did not have access to the results of the revolution in biology — genetic engineering — which began at that time. As far as is currently known, the recent Iraqi programme was not advanced enough to use such technology (although it was available in principle).

That, however, was not the case in the Soviet Union. The Soviet Union had had an interest in biological warfare research since the 1920s, and there was concern in the West about their capabilities during the early years of the Cold War. What has become apparent in recent years is that a decision was taken by the Soviet Union at the time of the agreement of the Biological and Toxin Weapons Convention in the early 1970s to initiate a massive offensive biological warfare programme. That something unusual was happening was first obvious to the public when information suggesting that a number of people had been killed by the accidental release of anthrax from a military facility in Sverdlovsk in 1979 became irrefutable.[67,68] A systematic account of the Soviet programme is not yet in the public domain, but the most comprehensive description concludes that the Soviet programme was an order of magnitude bigger than the US programme at its peak.[69] The question that arises is what could have been the objective of such a huge effort?

John Steinbrunner has recently suggested that it was connected with the problems the Soviet military thought they would encounter had they been tasked with invading Western

Europe. In his view, when President Nixon renounced biological weapons and the US argued that such weapons offered no useful advantages, the Soviet Union concluded, on the contrary, that they might have a central role.[70] He argues that the best guess from the available information is that these weapons would not have been used directly in battle against NATO forces, but in order to subdue the population's resistance to occupation. Ken Alibeck, a highly placed defector, has also suggested that in the event of war, large-scale biological attacks would have been made on US cities with multiple-warheaded missiles.[71]

What is important is the accumulating evidence that the Soviet Union was using modern means of genetic engineering in its offensive biological warfare programme — focusing on offensive research into such agents as anthrax, smallpox and bubonic plague. This suggests that it was in a different category from what had gone before — perhaps best regarded as a *third generation* programme of this century which could foreshadow events in the next. It will be convenient to return to this matter in detail in the next chapter, when the implications of developments in modern biology and medicine are analysed.

1990 to 1998 and beyond

The 1990-91 Gulf War was a significant event in the evolution of biological warfare. The renewed threat of biological warfare was taken very seriously. Considerable protective measures were taken by coalition forces against the threat of use of chemical and biological weapons. These protective measures could have been involved in the subsequent development of 'Gulf War Syndrome' amongst US and UK forces.[72] An examination of this issue is beyond the scope of this report, but clearly important lessons can be learned from research into this matter. Presently, the most important concern "is that biological weapons continue to pose a threat, particularly in conflicts involving Third World powers and/or terrorist groups".[73] These two possible sources of threat have certainly received considerable coverage in the strategic studies literature during the 1990s.[74]

An illustrative case of the temptation to initiate biological weapons programmes in conflict-prone regions of the world, involves the former apartheid regime in South Africa. Though the public record is presently unclear, it seems increasingly probable that diverse forms of biological weaponry were developed. Allegations which are currently being considered by the Truth and Reconciliation Commission focus on the work of Dr Wouter Basson, a cardiologist by training, who was reportedly involved in atrocities which included: distributing Mandrax tablets to black townships to pacify them, and developing infertility drugs to target the black population.[75] There have also been allegations that water supplies in neighbouring countries were deliberately contaminated with cholera and that biological weapons were used for political assassination. Undoubtedly, as these proceedings unfold, more details of these atrocities will emerge.

As for terrorist use of biological weapons,[76] it is fortunate that there are few known incidents to date, but there are good reasons to believe that bioterrorism could occur more frequently in the future as terrorists become more technologically sophisticated. For example, the Aum Shinrikyo sect in Japan, responsible for a Sarin nerve gas attack on the Tokyo subway in 1995, commanded the resources to develop weapons of mass destruction. Reports indicate that, in addition to the use of Sarin nerve gas, the sect:[77]

> *"...included among its members skilled scientists...who attempted to generate weapons using anthrax, botulinum toxin, Q-fever and even ebola..."*

Fortunately, again, the available evidence indicates that their efforts to use such weapons failed, possibly because of the difficulties involved in the effective dispersal of the agents. However, if a terrorist group were state-sponsored, the probability that it could use biological weapons successfully would certainly increase. Moreover, given a longer period of time to carry out its research, a large non-state-sponsored terrorist group might well be able to solve the engineering problems involved in dispersing a biological agent effectively.

With the increasing probability of terrorist use of biological weapons against civilian populations, there is renewed interest in the provision of low-cost civil defence measures. Civil defence against an all-out nuclear attack during the Cold War was widely seen as ineffective, but in the 'new world of mass destruction', where it can be argued that biological weapons — easy to produce and as effective as nuclear weapons — are the most important threat, effective civil defence could be important as a means of blunting the consequences of an attack.[78] Certainly, there is considerable medical knowledge available on the 'classical' biological warfare agents and of protective measures and treatment strategies against them, which can be used to limit their effectiveness.[79]

A typology of future biological warfare

In an effort to assist the process of thinking through the likely effectiveness of various means of strengthening the BTWC, Wheelis[80] proposed a three-point typology of biological warfare involving the nature of the aggressor, the scale of release of agent and the identity of the target (Table 2.7). Within each dimension of this typology Wheelis described three possibilities.

Table 2.7: Dimensions of biological warfare*

1. Nature of the aggressor		2. Scale of release of agent		3. Target	
(a)	Nations	(a)	Point source release	(a)	Humans
(b)	Subnational groups	(b)	Medium-scale release	(b)	Plants
(c)	Individuals	(c)	Large-scale release	(c)	Animals

*From[81]

He went on to produce a nine-cell matrix of possible types of biological warfare against humans by combining the nature of the aggressor with the scale of release of agent (Table 2.8).

Table 2.8: Types of biological warfare*

Scale of release of agent	Nature of aggressor		
	Individual	Subnational group	State
Point source	eg Criminal act	eg Assassination	eg Assassination
Medium scale	eg Criminal act	eg Terrorist	eg Military tactical
Large scale	Not possible	eg National liberation (army) use	eg Military strategic

*From[82]

Whilst it is not well known outside of specialist circles, the Rajneeshee sect contaminated the salad bars of ten restaurants in Oregon with *Salmonella typhimurium* in 1984 and made at least 750 people ill. This can be categorised as a medium-scale, terrorist attack by a sub-national group (ie the central cell of the matrix). Additionally, the cells of the matrix could also be grouped into three supercategories of *purpose*: terrorist or individual use; covert use; or military use. An example of covert use against agricultural resources would be the deliberate infection of the staple crops of another country in order to weaken its economy without the overt declaration of war.

Consideration of the brief history of biological warfare, just reviewed, suggests a number of other characteristics that might usefully be considered in a detailed typology of future biological warfare possibilities. The list of purposes that such warfare might be intended to serve could obviously be extended to include, for example, deterrence, or in a more extreme case, genocide. Slander by false accusation of the use of biological warfare is also

31

possible.[83] Moreover, a false accusation may be difficult to disprove and therefore very damaging to the accused state. In regard to Wheelis' original three-point typology (Table 2.8), it might also be useful to add 'material' to the potential targets in view of possible developments in the field of non-lethal warfare.[84] With the probable difference in degree of preparedness, it might be helpful as well to subdivide the 'human' category of target into civil and military, or even to add ethnic group.

Given the ubiquitous nature of biological warfare, it would be possible to further expand the typology developed by Wheelis — for example by considering the timescale of effects, which might perhaps be decades or generations. Moreover, much remains to be learned about the history of biological weapons programmes, eg of the unwitting involvement of civilian populations in germ warfare tests off the Dorset coast in the 1960s.[85] Such new information might also suggest modification of Wheelis' typology. We will return to this issue in later chapters, but an important question must first be addressed: to what extent might modern biology radically alter the whole problem of controlling biological warfare? We must ask whether the third generation offensive biological weapons programme could be succeeded by a *fourth*, or even a *fifth* level of sophistication.

Chapter 3

The impact of biotechnology

Having reviewed the history of biological warfare, and in particular its development during the last century as understanding of microbiology and pathogenesis has grown, we turn now to the potential impact of today's revolution in biotechnology. The entry on biological warfare in the *Encyclopedia of Microbiology* notes that the advent of genetic engineering has two potential impacts, the first on the offensive threat and the second on possible defence.[1] So while our main concern here is with the impact of modern biotechnology on the evolution of the threat, the more benign impact on the evolution of protection and defences should be kept in mind.

The potential impact of scientific and technological developments were a concern even before the Biological and Toxin Weapons Convention (BTWC) was agreed. In the difficult period in the early 1970s, when there was dispute over whether chemical and biological weapons should be treated together or in different disarmament conventions, the United Kingdom warned that there was a danger in delaying an agreement on biological weapons because of the rapid pace of scientific advances.[2] This was indeed prophetic because even though the two issues were separated, and the BTWC was agreed at that time, the Convention did not have adequate verification provisions to prevent the application of genetic engineering to offensive biological warfare programmes.

The BTWC and the biotechnology revolution

It is important to stress that technological developments do not necessarily lead to weapon systems development. Such a technological deterministic viewpoint would ignore the fact that social processes can enhance or restrict the application of any new technology.[3] The Biological and Toxin Weapons Convention, which entered into force in 1975, has a first article which defines the scope of the agreement. In defining what is covered by the Convention, Article I states:[4]

> *"Each State Party to this Convention undertakes never in any circumstances to develop, produce, stockpile or otherwise acquire or retain:*
>
> 1. *Microbial or other biological agents, or toxins whatever their origin or method of production, of types and in quantities that have no justification for prophylactic, protective or other peaceful purposes;*
>
> 2. *Weapons, equipment or means of delivery designed to use such agents or toxins for hostile purposes or in armed conflict."*

Article I.1 therefore embodies what has been called a 'General Purpose Criterion' of the same kind as is found in the recently agreed Chemical Weapons Convention (CWC). As Perry Robinson explained:[5]

> *"...The negotiators agreed language which defined the scope of the CWC as extending to* all *toxic chemicals, and to* all *chemicals from which any toxic chemical can be made* ('precursors'), *subject to the following proviso:* 'except

34

> where intended for purposes not prohibited under
> this Convention, as long as the types and quantities
> are consistent with such purposes'..."

Whilst the process of implementation of the CWC is still in its early stages and some issues remain to be resolved, the CWC does spell out in some detail what is presently prohibited and what is not. This gives considerable definition to the 'General Purpose Criterion'. In the BTWC, agreed twenty years earlier:

> *"...The corresponding language...brings within the scope of*
> *that treaty all* 'microbial or other biological agents, or
> toxins whatever their origin or method of
> production, of types and in quantities that have no
> justification for prophylactic, protective or other
> peaceful purposes'."

However, the BTWC does not spell out what is and what is not prohibited in the way the CWC does, and it does not contain the very effective verification mechanism of the CWC. Indeed, Article V of the BTWC has been slightingly called a substitute for a verification provision rather than a verification clause by one commentator.[6]

The General Purpose Criterion of the BTWC is nevertheless a sweeping prohibition. Clearly, by prohibiting *purposes* rather than *things* the agreement covers any future developments besides the possibilities known at the time it was agreed. Additionally, Article XII of the Convention allows for five-yearly reviews to assess the operation of the BTWC (Table 3.1).

The results of these Review Conferences are embodied in Final Declarations and no state can ignore the results of the reviews which have legal standing in defining what has been agreed. We can thus follow the developing concerns and actions of the States Parties from the Final Declarations of the Review Conferences. More than that, in regard to the scope of the BTWC set out in Article I, we can follow in detail the concerns about the

Table 3.1: Review Conferences of the Biological and Toxin Weapons Convention

Signed	1972
Entered into force	1975
First Review Conference	1980
Second Review Conference	1986
Third Review Conference	1991
Fourth Review Conference	1996
No. of States now party to the Convention	140

growing impact of biotechnology from the scientific background papers provided by States Parties for the Review Conferences.

Biotechnology, of course, has a long history of use in the brewing, baking, dairy and other industries. However, over the last few decades, the rapid advances in molecular biology have resulted in the ability to interchange DNA of different organisms.[7] The background to the Five Year Review Conferences of the BTWC, therefore, has been one of enormous developments in technological capabilities, as discoveries made in research laboratories have been put to commercial use, particularly in the pharmaceutical industry.[8] It is also probable that we are only in the first phase of a revolution in biology which will be a major element in the growth of the world economy in the next century.

Running parallel to the increasingly active development of modern biotechnology over the last 35 years, there have been efforts to understand, classify and regulate the civil use of micro-organisms that might affect humans, animals, plants or the environment.[9] The development of such civil regulatory systems can be expected to continue around the world as the dangers are further clarified. Those interested in using diseases deliberately for malign purposes[10] would naturally be concerned with the higher-risk organisms. A listing of potential agents in a Russian official paper[11] illustrates just how wide the range of possibilities could be (Table 3.2).

Table 3.2: Illustrative list of potential BW agents*

"BACTERIA, RICKETTSIA, CHLAMYDIA, FUNGI, VIRUSES:

Yersinia pestis, Bacillus anthracis, Pseudomonas mallei, Pseudomonas pseudomallei, Francisella tularensis, Brucella melitensis, Vibrio cholerae, Legionella pneumophilia... [30 in total]

TOXINS OF MICROORGANISMS:

Botulinum toxins, enterotoxin A *Staphylococcus aureus*, alpha-toxin *Staphylococcus aureus*, neurotoxin *Shigella dysenteriae*;

TOXINS OF ANIMAL ORIGIN:

Tetrodotoxin, conotoxins, batrachotoxin;

TOXINS OF PLANTS AND SEAWEED TOXINS:

Abrin, ricin, saxitoxin;

TOXINS OF SNAKES AND SPIDERS:

Taipoxin, textilotoxin...[11 in total]

NEUROPEPTIDES:

Endothelin..."

---

*From[12]

The BTWC review conferences

For the first Five Year Review Conference of the BTWC in 1980 the three Depositary States appointed to take overall responsibility for the Convention — the USSR, US and UK — produced a joint paper on *New Scientific and Technological Developments* which were relevant to the Convention.[13] The paper clearly identified the key scientific discovery by which recombinant DNA techniques permitted "the transfer of genetic material between widely divergent species" and acknowledged that important industrial applications of the new technology were envisaged. It also accepted that the new technology might be misused to modify existing organisms to make them more suitable for use in various ways in warfare. However, the paper concluded that:

"Although recombinant DNA techniques could facilitate genetic manipulation of micro-organisms for biological and toxin weapon purposes, the resulting agents are unlikely to have advantages over known natural agents sufficient to provide compelling new motives for illegal production and military use in the foreseeable future..."

This relatively sanguine viewpoint also appears to underlie the Final Declaration of the Conference, which in regard to Article I, noted that:[14]

"The Conference believes that Article I has proved sufficiently comprehensive to have covered recent scientific and technological developments relevant to the Convention."

The 'foreseeable future' noted in the background paper on scientific and technological developments by the Depositary States, however, turned out to be very short indeed.

The background papers on scientific and technological developments produced for the Review Conferences would have drawn on reports produced within the various State administrations. The first impact of the new technology was clearly to increase production capabilities. Genes for required products (such as insulin) could be inserted into microorganisms and these could then be grown in large quantities under controlled conditions. As early as 1981 a US report, *Recombinant DNA and the Biological Warfare Threat*, drew attention to this possible new means of cheaply manufacturing toxins.[15] The point was elaborated further in a 1985 US report, *Implications of Present Knowledge and Past Experience for a Possible Future Chemical/Conventional Conflict*, which suggested that:[16]

"The most potent toxins are proteins themselves. It is likely that their utilization as warfare agents can be greatly enhanced by molecular biology and genetic engineering.... Modifications to the toxin to increase stability and/or toxicity

*are made by isolating the gene...for the toxin. This toxin
gene can then be altered....When the desired toxin is
achieved, it can be inexpensively produced in large
quantities using genetic engineering techniques."*

It is little wonder, then, that the Final Declaration of the
Second Review Conference in 1986 specifically pointed out that
Article I applied to toxins:[17]

*"The Conference reaffirms that the Convention
unequivocally applies to all natural or artificially created
microbial or other biological agents or toxins whatever their
origin or method of production. Consequently, toxins (both
proteinaceous and non-proteinaceous) of a microbial,
animal or vegetable nature and their synthetically produced
analogues are covered."*

At this time the States Parties also began to try to improve
transparency in relation to the BTWC by agreeing a series of
annual data exchanges known as 'Confidence Building Measures'.
Though confirmed and developed at the Third Review
Conference in 1991, these have not been widely regarded as a
success.[18]

The process of scientific analysis of the impact of modern
biotechnology, and updating of Article I, have continued through
the third and fourth Five Year Review Conferences of the
BTWC.[19,20,21,22] As concerns have increased, very detailed studies
have been made within, and in association with, the military
establishments of various countries.[23,24] The general thrust of
conclusions has been much less sanguine than that of the
Depositary States in 1980. The UK, for example, concluded in
1991 that:[25]

*"There can thus be no doubt that the proliferation of
legitimate civilian industrial microbiology activities, and
the continuing development of the underlying theory and
equipment, has increased the potential worldwide for*

> *developing and producing biological weapons in*
> *contravention of the BWC..."*

The Final Declaration of the Third Review Conference in 1991 thus repeated the view of the Second Review Conference in stating:[26]

> *"The Conference, conscious of apprehensions arising from relevant scientific and technological developments,* inter alia, *in the fields of microbiology, genetic engineering and biotechnology and the possibilities of their use for purposes inconsistent with the objectives and the provisions of the Convention, reaffirms that the undertaking given by the States parties in Article I applies to all such developments..."*

In the following sentence the words "or altered" were added to the wording (see above) from the Final Declaration of the Second Review Conference. This now read:

> *"...The Conference also reaffirms that the Convention unequivocally covers all microbial or other biological agents or toxins, naturally or artificially created* or altered, *whatever their origin or method of production."* [emphasis added]

This addition clearly reiterated that genetically engineered organisms were covered by the BTWC. In addition to attempting to enhance the 'Confidence Building Measures' agreed at the previous review, the States Parties in 1991 also agreed to undertake a scientific analysis of the possibilities for verifying the BTWC in what became known as the VEREX process. This led on, through the Special Conference of States Parties in 1994, to current efforts to strengthen the Convention[27] through a legally-binding instrument (a Verification Protocol) that will be discussed in Chapter 5.

Prior to the 1991 Third Review Conference, the Canadian Government issued a special study, *Novel Toxins and Bioregulators,* which drew attention to the difficulties that these might cause for verification of the BTWC.[28] The background papers on scientific and technological developments prepared by the United States, in 1991 and again in 1996,[29] drew attention to the potential problems that could arise from the misuse of natural or modified bioregulatory peptides. Significantly, the report argued:

> *"Their range of activity covers the entire living system, from mental processes (eg endorphins) to many aspects of health such as control of mood, consciousness, temperature control, sleep or emotions, exerting regulatory effects on the body. Even a small imbalance in these natural substances could have serious consequences, inducing fear, fatigue, depression or incapacitation. These substances would be extremely difficult to detect, but could cause serious consequences or even death if used improperly."*

Such concerns were reflected in the Final Declaration of the Fourth Review Conference by the further addition of the wording "as well as their components" to the paragraph developed in 1986 and 1991. This now read:[30]

> *"The Conference also reaffirms that the Convention unequivocally covers all microbial or other biological agents or toxins, naturally or artificially created or altered, as well as their components, whatever their origin or method of production, of types and in quantities that have no justification for prophylactic, protective or other peaceful purposes."*

This wording obviously also covered the increasing capabilities for using fragments of toxins, as understanding of their mechanisms of action grew.[31] Clearly, one major aspect of the growth of modern biology has been the increasing understanding of receptor mechanisms in neuroscience and of how to target chemicals at such receptors.[32]

It would be difficult to argue, though, that the central feature of modern biotechnology in the 1990s was anything other than the Human Genome Project.[33] The British background paper for the 1996 Fourth Review Conference made the point:[34]

> *"It is predicted that the human genome will be sequenced by the year 2005. The information is expected to lead to radical new treatments for a broad range of human disease..."*

Yet the paper continued:

> *"...It cannot be ruled out that information from such genetic research could be considered for the design of weapons targeted against specific ethnic or racial groups..."*

This specific possibility will be considered in the next chapter, but it may be noted here that the 1996 Review Conference clearly took the potential misuse of knowledge of the human genome very seriously, and modified its earlier statement on apprehensions arising from scientific developments to read:[35]

> *"The Conference, conscious of apprehensions arising from relevant scientific and technological developments,* inter alia, *in the fields of microbiology, biotechnology, molecular biology, genetic engineering and any applications resulting from genome studies, and the possibilities of their use for purposes inconsistent with the objectives and the provisions of the Convention, reaffirms that the undertaking given by the States Parties in Article I applies to all such developments."*

The newly-added words "molecular biology" and "any applications resulting from genome studies" clearly reflect the concern that such new capabilities might be misused.

By the end of the Cold War period the range of potential chemical weapons and biological weapons had been considerably extended, and had been classifed in an emerging spectrum of threat.[36] This spectrum is set out in Table 3.3.

Table 3.3: The CBW Spectrum*

Chemicals

Classical CW
  Mustard gas
  Nerve gas

Emerging CW
  Toxic industrial chemicals
  Toxic pharmaceutical chemicals
  Toxic agricultural chemicals

Bioregulators
  Peptides

Toxins
  Saxitoxin
  Mycotoxin
  Ricin

Biological organisms

Genetically manipulated BW
  Modified/tailored bacteria, viruses

Traditional BW
  Bacteria
  Viruses
  Rickettsia

*From[37]

But concerns about the impact of genetic engineering[38] were little understood by those outside of professional defence circles until information on the Soviet offensive biological weapons programme became available to the general public.

The Soviet offensive BW programme

Information on the Soviet programme appears to have come mainly from two high-level defectors, Dr Pasechnik who came to the UK in 1989 and Dr Alibekov (Alibeck) who arrived in the United States in 1992. Some of the information they provided has entered the public domain, most recently in a television programme[39] and articles[40,41] featuring Dr Alibeck. Whilst this material does not provide a full, coherent account of the massive programme carried out over two decades, it does show quite clearly that the first fruits of the revolution in modern biology were applied to the development of new weapons. We can therefore regard it as different in kind — a *third generation* programme — from what had gone before. In what could be a repeat of earlier misperceptions (see Chapter 2) which led to the initiation of offensive biological warfare programmes,[42] there is evidence that the Soviet upper echelons doubted the US renunciation of its own offensive biological weapons programme in 1969.[43,44,45] Nevertheless, the Soviet programme was in total contradiction to their obligations under the BTWC.

Despite the fact that the organisation was partly involved in civil activities, the first feature that is striking about the Soviet programme, initiated in 1973 directly after the BTWC was signed, is its scale. According to Alibeck:[46]

> "...At its height, 32,000 people worked for Biopreparat (the civilian pharmaceutical and vaccine company that served as a cover for biological weapons work), an additional 10,000 or so worked in Defence Ministry bioweapons laboratories, and thousands of others were scattered through other agencies."

Biopreparat had some forty research and production sites, at least twelve of these facilities being on an 'enormous' scale.[47] The second striking feature is the amount, and types, of agents produced. Again according to Alibeck:[48]

> *"The Soviets had the capacity to produce huge amounts of many different agents. The hundreds of tons of anthrax and dozens of tons of smallpox and plague that the Soviets kept stockpiled could be loaded into bombs and missiles for use within days."*

As noted in the previous chapter, these agents appear to have been intended for very large-scale use in Europe, and in the United States, in the event of major war.

Alibeck has claimed that advanced molecular biology research related to biological warfare is still going on in Russia,[49] but some of his claims are doubted by informed US scientists.[50] What is clear, however, is that the third striking feature of the Soviet programme is the use of genetic engineering. Dr Pasechnik, the first senior defector, had been director of the Institute of Ultrapure Biopreparations in Leningrad. The institute was doing offensive research on *Yersinia pestis*, the causative agent of plague. Richard Preston is one of a number of sources who make the same point:[51]

> *"...Natural plague is curable with antibiotics. After listening to Dr Pasechnik, the British concluded that the Soviet Union had developed a genetically engineered strain of plague that was resistant to antibiotics..."*

References to other sources are to be found in a recent review of potential threats from the deliberate misuse of disease in the next century.[52] It can only be hoped that current efforts to apply all of the accumulated Russian expertise to peaceful purposes are successful.[53]

The threat today

There is a multitude of ways in which biological agents might be misused. In military parlance[54] such concepts of use (COU) can be grouped into four general types: superpower *vs* superpower; state *vs* state; state *vs* factional element or *vice versa*; and terrorist use.

Clearly, considering the first of these types, huge-scale potential use of biological weapons by two antagonistic superpowers is no longer envisaged. Yet it is clear that we are in a period of considerable instability in the world system, where local and regional wars are frequent, and interventions by outside forces are likely to continue.[55] We should, therefore, be particularly concerned with the capabilities of states' biological weapons. In state *vs* state interactions:[56]

> "...personnel of strategic facilities, eg ports, airbases, command posts etc, could be targets during a tactical situation. Tactical applications against selected groups of unprotected troops by an unexpected attack can be envisaged..."

It is possible to see a reorientation towards dealing with such threats in the US today.[57] One scenario, given in public versions of a report entitled *Assessment of the Impact of Chemical and Biological Weapons on Joint Operations in 2010*, envisaged an attack with a cholera aerosol on supply ships *en route* to a theatre of war. The report suggested:[58]

> "If, for example, the attack was [with] a microencapsulated agent — which will survive long-term — the...crews would not become ill for a few days.... At that point...the so-called 'plague convoy' would be unlikely to be granted port rights..."

A key finding of the report, therefore, was that such an attack could have a major impact on operations. Interruption of supply was a more likely threat than direct battlefield use of biological weapons. What is of particular interest here is the reference to 'microencapsulation' of the cholera agent. Microencapsulation is the process of encasing a substance within a thin protective shell — a physical process widely used in commercial industry since the

1920s. It has offensive military applications in enhancing the resistance of agents to environmental degradation and making detection and identification more difficult.[59]

This does raise the question of the extent to which genetic engineering might now also be used to 'tailor' agents in specific ways for other purposes that states might require in the new strategic situation. In short, if the Soviet third generation programme (for a superpower *vs* superpower context) is now over, what might arise in a *fourth generation* programme designed for a state *vs* state context? That these are not just theoretical issues was re-emphasised by the decision taken late in 1997 to vaccinate *all* US military personnel against anthrax.[60] The idea that genetic engineering might allow agents to be designed for particular purposes has been clearly understood for some time, as is clear from documents of the early 1980s.[61,62] What is different now is the underlying advance in civil science and technology that has been made.[63] As a British civil scientist noted, in a presentation to a security studies seminar:[64]

> "...it is important to realise that, as our knowledge of the molecular mechanisms of microbial pathogenesis increases, it will become possible to modify pathogenicity using much more subtle changes..."

He illustrated his point by suggesting that:

> "...Modifications to a micro-organism which change the way it might interact with the immune system, or alter its tissue tropism or interaction with certain host enzymes, may profoundly alter its pathogenic potential..."

Such changes, he argued, could "provide a route to the tailoring of micro-organisms for BW purposes". This knowledge, for example, could be used to dramatically increase the lethality of human influenza.[65]

The technical annex to the US Secretary of State's report in late 1997, *Proliferation: Threat and Response*,[66] points out that, while classical agents developed in earlier programmes remain the greatest concern and while, historically, it has been difficult to accentuate a particular character of an agent in a controlled way:

> *"...Advances in biotechnology, genetic engineering, and related scientific fields provide increasing potential to control more of these factors, possibly leading to the ability to use biological warfare agents as tactical battlefield weapons."*

The potential types of novel agents that the report suggests could be produced are set out in Table 3.4.

Table 3.4: Novel agents that could be produced by genetic engineering*

"- Benign microorganisms, genetically altered to produce a toxin, venom, or bioregulator.

- Microorganisms resistant to antibiotics, standard vaccines, and therapeutics.

- Microorganisms with enhanced aerosol and environmental stability.

- Immunologically-altered microorganisms able to defeat standard identification, detection, and diagnostic methods.

- Combinations of the above four types with improved delivery systems."

* From[67]

What is very significant is the accent put on the coming capabilities to control, ie tailor micro-organisms for particular purposes. Following the listing given in Table 3.4 the annex continues:

> *"It is noteworthy that each of these techniques seeks to capitalise on the extreme lethality, virulence, or infectivity of biological warfare agents and exploit this potential by developing methods to deliver more efficiently and to control these agents on the battlefield."*

It is certainly not difficult to find possible examples in the open literature. For example, in a 1983 US report it was argued that:[68]

> *"Genetic manipulation to modify the effect of environmental factors such as exposure to ultraviolet light, temperature, pH tolerance etc, could be used to modify organism survival under specific conditions. For example, spore-forming organisms such as* B. anthracis *could be given coding to produce a less protective spore which would decrease the classical persistency of the spores."*

In short, anthrax could be used as a weapon without the problem of having long-term contamination of the environment after it had killed its victims.

Today there is, of course, a perfectly legitimate international study underway of the *Bacillus subtilis* genome,[69] and numerous investigations of the mechanism of sporulation.[70] One author, whose reseach was in part supported by the US Army Research Office, noted in a recent review entitled *Mechanisms for the Prevention of Damage to DNA in Spores of Bacillus Species* that small acid-soluble α/β-type proteins were very important in protecting the spore DNA from environmental damage.[71] The genes for the major small acid-soluble proteins have been cloned and deletion mutations without either α or β (α–β–) genes have been constructed:

> *"...Strikingly,* α–β– *spores are much more sensitive than wild-type spores to UV radiation, heat, oxidizing agents and freeze-drying, although the spores' [gamma]-radiation resistance is the same..."*

Whilst the work reported is for *Bacillus subtilis* the author notes that "the mechanisms ensuring DNA protection in dormant *B. subtilis* spores probably also operate in spores of other *Bacillus* species, as well as in spores of *Clostridium* species". Thus the idea put forward in 1983 might now be achieved through genetic engineering. Of course, an understanding of sporulation and germination of such spore-forming bacteria could also perhaps allow the development of better means of protection against the misuse of biological warfare agents. However, it is not necessary to refer to theoretical dangers. In 1997 it was reported that the US Defense Advanced Research Projects Agency (DARPA) had been funded $60 million to develop countermeasures of a revolutionary kind against pathogens. The report stated that:[72]

> *"The initiative stems mainly from concern over the potential for genetically engineered biological pathogens to be used against US troops or in a terrorist scenario."*

Senior DARPA officials were reported as saying that:

> *"...the Japanese Aum Shinrikyo cult successfully reengineered an e-coli agent to 'place' botulinum toxin 'inside' the original agent."*

The report stated that the sect had not deployed the genetically engineered agent, but their goal was to:

> *"...develop a reengineered agent in which the highly lethal component would not affect the victims for some time."*

It is known that concern over possible terrorist use of biological weapons is common amongst high-level US officials, including the President, and that much effort has been expended to improve protection for the population in the event of an attack. Yet in one recent exercise in which a terrorist was assumed to have used a genetically modified smallpox-Marburg virus combination many deficiencies were revealed.[73]

If the tailoring of known agents is the major concern of the near future, what of the somewhat longer term? The Technical Annex to *Proliferation: Threat and Response* suggests that long-term threats are not easily predicted, but presents a set of technological trends that could be of significance. These are given in Table 3.5.

Table 3.5: Significant trends related to future biological weapons possibilities*

"- Genetically engineered vectors in the form of modified infectious organisms will be increasingly employed as tools in medicine and the techniques will become more widely available.

- Strides will be made in understanding of infectious disease mechanisms and in microbial genetics that are responsible for disease processes.

- An increased understanding of the human immune system function and disease mechanisms will shed light on the circumstances that cause individual susceptibility to infectious disease.

- Vaccines and antidotes will be improved over the long term, perhaps to the point where classical biological warfare agents will offer less utility as a means of causing casualties."

*From[74]

Obviously, many malign possibilities could arise when scientific work being carried out in laboratories today eventually results in usable technologies two or three decades in the future.[75,76] Those who wish to prevent the further development and proliferation of biological weapons, therefore, need to have a sense of what could happen later — say in *fifth generation* offensive biological weapons programmes in the early decades of the twenty-first century — as they consider what should be done today. One often-mentioned possibility, of weapons specifically targeted at particular ethnic groups, is considered in the next chapter.

Chapter 4

Genetic weapons

It has been suggested that attacks on specific ethnic groups are amongst the possible future uses of biological weapons. No such possibility would arise if different ethnic groups did not frequently come into conflict. As Klaus Larres noted in his review of W R Polk's *Neighbours and Strangers: The Fundamentals of Foreign Affairs*, our strategies for dealing with foreigners range from isolation through accommodation to extermination.[1] Genocide — the intended destruction in whole, or in part, of a national, ethnic, racial or religious group — is not an infrequent occurrence in human history. There have been many recent attempts at genocide. The victims have included the Kurds in Iraq, Tutsi in Rwanda and the people of East Timor.[2] Little wonder then that the Genocide Convention,[3] which came into force in 1951 after the terrible genocides of the Second World War (Table 4.1), had some 120 States Parties by 1995.

However, genocide is a continual possibility in a world characterised by vast differences in wealth, subject to environmental limits on growth and full of weaponry.[5]

Types of genetic weapons

It will be recalled that the UK contribution to the background paper on new scientific and technological developments for the

Fourth Review Conference of the BTWC in 1996 stated that the knowledge arising from the Human Genome Project (HGP):[6]

> "...*could be considered for the design of weapons targeted against specific ethnic or racial groups...*"

Consideration of ethnic-specific biological weapons, however, long predated the advent of the Human Genome Project.

Table 4.1: The Genocide Convention*

Article 2. In the present Convention, genocide means any of the following acts committed with intent to destroy, in whole or in part, a national, ethnical, racial or religious group, as such:

    (a)   Killing members of the group;

    (b)   Causing serious bodily or mental harm to members of the group...

Article 3. The following acts shall be punishable:

    (a)   Genocide;

    (b)   Conspiracy to commit genocide;

    (c)   Direct and public incitement to commit genocide;

    (d)   Attempt to commit genocide;

    (e)   Complicity in genocide...

*From[4]

The use of smallpox against the American Indians centuries ago (Chapter 2) was almost certainly a deliberate military act. Moreover, it can hardly be argued that we have now advanced so far morally that an ethnic-specific weapon would not be used today if it became available during a severe conflict between two deeply antagonistic groups. Early in the development of the US offensive biological weapons programme Colonel Creasy, Chief of Research and Engineering of the US Chemical Corps, suggested that one factor favouring the potentialities of anti-personnel biological warfare was that, "[a]gents may be selected because of known susceptibility of the target population".[7] This leaves little doubt that using the differential susceptibility of different populations to various diseases had been considered at that time.

It is not essential to focus on the genetic constitution of a particular group in order to attack it specifically. Clearly, vaccination of the attacker against the intended biological agent would give specificity if the target population was not vaccinated. Attacking a particular population with lethal toxins could achieve the same effect.[8] Despite such possibilities, however, most discussion of ethnic-specific weapons has centred on what are termed 'genetic' weapons, which involve the attempt to target genetic differences between ethnic groups.

Genetic weapons are clearly an emotive issue and have long been the subject of vocal claims of wrongdoing[9,10] and counter-claims of false accusation.[11] Moreover, even in regard to the possibilities that may be opened up by the Human Genome Project, the UK was careful to add a reservation to its warning, concerning the possible misuse of new knowledge to produce weapons targeted against specific groups, by stating:[12]

> *"...it is far from clear that the development of such weapons could ever be anything more than a theoretical possibility..."*

What causes alarm today, however, is that warnings are coming not only from the medical community (see Chapter 1), but also from other credible sources — there have been indications, for example, that the US Secretary of Defense is concerned about the possible development of genetic weapons. In June 1997 *Jane's Defence Weekly* reported that Secretary Cohen[13] "quoted other reports about what he called 'certain types of pathogens that would be ethnic specific so that they could just eliminate certain ethnic groups and races'". Then, after a later interview with the Defense Secretary in August 1997 it was stated that[14] "[h]e also continued to insist that the science community is 'very close' to being able to manufacture 'genetically engineered pathogens that could be ethnically specific'". It is difficult to imagine that a top government official would have made such a statement without careful consideration. What then are the scientific facts which might have caused the Secretary of Defense to be concerned?

Prediction of genetic weapons

In accounts during the 1980s of the possible development of genetic weapons,[15,16,17] a frequent source of scientific data was a paper by Carl A Larson, published in the journal *Military Review* in November 1970.[18] At that time Larson was head of the Department of Human Genetics at the Institute of Genetics, University of Lund, Sweden. As holder of that position, his analysis had to be given some weight. Its credibility in military circles was probably also enhanced by the fact that the journal *Military Review* was published by the US Army Command and General Staff College at Fort Leavenworth, Kansas.

Larson's paper, in fact, was mainly concerned with the possible development of a new range of chemical weapons, including incapacitants. Individual differences in response to chemical agents had been known about for some time, but Larson reviewed what was known of differences between *populations* in reaction to drugs. He clearly saw the basis of such population differences as genetic:

> *"Scores of enzyme failures due to gene mutations have now become known....The study of such heritable disturbances has included their prevalence in different geographical regions."*

Nevertheless, the overall impression is that Larson was pointing to possible future developments rather than near-term practical possibilities. The question is whether, almost 30 years later, genetic weapons have become a practical possibility.

There does not appear to have been detailed consideration by reputable scientists in the open literature of the application of modern biotechnology to the possible construction of genetic weapons until the 1990s. Then in 1992 the widely read specialist journal *Defense News* carried a report which noted a scientist arguing that genetic engineering may enable us to:[19]

> "...recognize DNA from different people and attach different things that will kill only that group of people.... You will be able to determine the difference between blacks and whites and Orientals and Jews and Swedes and Finns and develop an agent that will kill only [a particular] group."

Thus the threat would appear to have become very much more of a practical proposition.

Such arguments have been set out at greatest length in an appendix to the 1993 Stockholm Peace Research Institute's *Yearbook*.[20] The authors of the appendix were Bo Rybeck, Director General of the Swedish National Defence Research Establishment and a former Surgeon General of the Swedish Armed Forces, Professor Tamas Bartfai, head of the Department of Neurochemistry and Neurotoxicology at the University of Stockholm, and Dr S J Lundin, former Senior Director of Research of the Swedish National Defence Research Establishment. The appendix is entitled "Benefits and threats of developments in biotechnology and genetic engineering," but the authors' main concern is evident in the opening two paragraphs where, after noting the potential benefits of the large-scale application of the new technology, they continued:

> "...While modern biotechniques are revolutionizing medicine and agriculture, the possibility exists of their misuse for political ends, for clandestine production and refinement of biological weapons (BW), and for future development of weapons of mass extermination which could be used for genocide."

Specifically, in the view of these eminent authors:

> "Such a weapon system has not yet been developed, but the speed of scientific and technical progress is such that early

57

> *warnings of potential misuse are justified. There are*
> *rumours and allegations of the development of sophisticated*
> *biological and toxin weapons and perhaps genetic weapons*
> *and of the techniques which could be used to create such*
> *weapons...*"

Particular mention is then made of the possible misuse of knowledge gained from the Human Genome Project and knowledge about genetic diversity.

These authors saw the possible misuse of new biotechnology in the production of genetic weapons as part of the potential impact of the new technology. The part of their argument of central importance here, however, is contained in the last sub-section of section VI where they ask quite directly, "Can 'genetic weapons' be developed?". Their answer is that if:

> "*...investigations provide sufficient data on ethnic genetic*
> *differences between population groups, it may be possible to*
> *use such data to target suitable micro-organisms to attack*
> *known receptor sites for which differences exist at a cell*
> *membrane level or even to target DNA sequences inside cells*
> *by viral vectors...*"

Then they point out that:

> "*...techniques to selectively kill targeted cells, inactivate*
> *specific DNA sequences, insert new sequences at selected*
> *points, and the like are rapidly being developed for several*
> *medical therapies, most importantly for gene therapy...*"

Whilst they note that ethnic differences do not match political borders well, and therefore "[i]t might be necessary for a user of genetic weapons to take risks with regard to his own and friendly populations", there can be little doubt that these authors see the development of genetic weapons as a significant risk.

Their argument can be broken down into three parts. As would be expected from the central importance of the Human

Genome Project for sequencing the whole of human DNA, they suggest first that the aim of the Human Genome Organisation (HUGO) is (Section II) to:

> "...*provide insight into the organisation and function of genetic material and in the course of this work to base physiology and medicine on solid molecular foundations...*"

We will therefore not just know the *structure* of the genome but, increasingly, we will understand how it works — its *function*. Clearly, with such knowledge it would be theoretically possible to interfere, in a benign or malign way, with the mechanism's operation.

Secondly, they note the clear genetic differences beween human groups and suggest that:

> "...*These genetic differences may in many cases be sufficiently large and stable so as to possibly be exploited by using naturally occurring, selective agents or by genetically engineering organisms and toxins with selectivity for an intended genetic marker...*"

Furthermore, they argue that as most of the genome does *not* code for proteins, since the genes appear to be separated by long lengths of DNA with no presently known function:

> "*When HUGO provides data on all protein-coding sequences and moreover on all non-protein-coding sequences the number of well defined genetic differences will increase dramatically compared to those known today...*"

The authors also point out that the use of DNA fingerprinting in forensic science requires analysis of the probability of particular sequences being from one individual and that such work may make it possible to distinguish sequences characteristic of particular groups. Moreover, this work is being done with large human groups in major areas of the population. The Human

Diversity Project, attempting to collect and store genetic material from 500 populations which may soon disappear, is also noted and would clearly supplement the growing knowledge of human genetic diversity. Thirdly and finally, the authors argue that:

> *"...A...number of illnesses seem to depend on the malfunction or lack of function of only one gene. In such cases gene therapy has been devised, implying the introduction of the correct gene to direct the production of a functional protein* in vivo *in the proper cells and tissues..."*

Furthermore:

> *"...The most recent versions of gene therapy use* in vivo *methods to introduce genes by viral vectors (and even by liposomes via the lungs). Gene therapy thus constitutes a major driving force in the development of efficient* in vivo *vectors (viral vectors, which can be misused to deliver harmful material such as so-called antisense oligonucleotides and ribozymes)."*

In short, if there are distinguishing DNA sequences between groups, and these can be targeted in a way that is known to produce a harmful outcome, a genetic weapon is possible. Whilst the likelihood of a theoretical weapon being turned into a practical system, and particularly over what timescale, is unstated, the theoretical possibility does seem to warrant further analysis. Each aspect of the argument will be considered in turn.

The Human Genome Project

The Human Genome Project began formally in 1990 as an international attempt to discover all of the human genes and make them available for further study.[21] At least 18 countries have established genome research projects and about 1,000 individuals from 50 countries are members of the Human Genome

Organisation, which helps to co-ordinate the international collaboration. The genomes of a number of other 'model' organisms are also being investigated. These range from the bacterium *Escherichia coli* through to the laboratory mouse.

The project was designed as a three-stage programme to produce genetic maps, physical maps and finally a complete nucleotide sequence. By April 1998 about 6,000 genes had been mapped to particular chromosomes and tens of thousands of gene fragments had been identified and were being assigned positions on chromosome maps. The aim of the physical mapping is to establish markers every 100,000 bases along each chromosome. This would require about 30,000 markers. As of the summer of 1997 about 8,000 landmarks were featured on the most complete map. An article in *Science* in late 1996 stated:[22]

> *"Central to the description of an organism's genome is a comprehensive catalog of the sequence and location of all its genes. Gene maps are now available for those organisms whose complete genomic sequence has been determined, including 141 viruses, 51 organelles, two eubacteria, one archeon, and one eukaryote (the yeast,* Saccharomyces cerevisiae)..."

The article was accompanied by an illustrative map of the human chromosomes with the position of various genes, which indicated what the eventual outcome of the Human Genome Project would look like in structural terms. By April 1998 some 2.5% of the human genome had been sequenced, but a great deal of progress had been made in developing automatic sequencing, and there appeared to be widespread confidence that the 2005 target date for completion of the project would be met.[23]

In 1996 Eric Lander asked what should follow on from that success. He argued that the Human Genome Project should be seen as this century's version of the discovery and consolidation of the periodic table by chemists in the last century:[24]

> *"The Human Genome Project aims to produce biology's periodic table — not 100 elements, but 100,000 genes; not a rectangle reflecting electron valences, but a tree structure depicting ancestral and functional affinities among the human genes..."*

He then set out ten goals for the next phase of research after 2005 (Table 4.2), in summary suggesting that "[t]he challenge ahead is to turn the periodic table produced by the era of structural genomics into tools for the coming era of functional genomics". Whilst Lander predicted that much more sophisticated tools will be needed for that task, the way ahead is not hard to discern from reviews of current research.[25]

Table 4.2: Goals for the Human Genome Project after 2005*

1. Routine re-sequencing of multi-megabase regions of human and mouse DNA.
2. Systematic identification of all common variants in human genes.
3. Rapid de novo sequencing from other organisms.
4. Simultaneous monitoring of the expression of all genes.
5. Generic tools for manipulating cell circuitry.
6. Monitoring the level and modification state of all proteins.
7. Systematic catalogs of protein interactions.
8. Identification of all basic protein shapes.
9. Increased attention to ethical, legal and social issues.
10. Public education.

*From[26]

Human genetic diversity

Social anthropologists[27] and biological anthropologists[28] have long argued that it is simplistic as well as dangerous to talk in terms of distinct human races. The Human Genome Project confirms that we have a series of genes placed along each of our 23 pairs of chromosomes, each gene of which, at a particular locus, may occur in different forms or alleles. The well-known ABO blood groups, discovered early this century, were throughly investigated because of their importance in blood transfusion.[29] Since there are more than two alleles of the determining gene, the ABO system is an example of genetic polymorphism. An individual's blood group is determined in a fairly straightforward way from the genotype, and the different frequencies of the alleles can be quite significant between different populations.[30] It may perhaps sometimes be convenient to use races and ethnicity as a form of shorthand, but the fundamental units of the human species are not races. The point is that:[31]

> *"...populations differ from one another in the frequencies of the same alleles they carry, and this can be used to group human populations by genetic similarity. Like morphological differences across the human species, these groupings are generally obvious when* extremes *are contrasted..." [emphasis added]*

Races do not exist but are social categories superimposed on these gradients of change in allele frequencies produced by the micro-evolution of our species as it spread across the globe.[32] Such gradients of change result from groups having slightly different genetic constitutions and from local adaptations in populations living in different environmental conditions. A well-known example is the adaptation to malaria through the high frequency of sickle cell anaemia found in populations in West Africa.[33]

It is also clear that the vast majority of variation in the human species is to be found within groups rather than between groups:[34]

> *"...If some catastrophic event were to occur so that only Norwegians, for example, were left on the face of the earth, close to 86% of total human genetic variation would still be preserved by them..."*

A number of our hominid relatives have disappeared, and we lack the genetic diversity of either the chimpanzees or the gorillas today. A possible explanation for this lack of diversity is that we all derive from a relatively small group of founders of our species:[35]

> *"...it may well be the case that the present [low] level of genetic diversity in our species dates to the emergence of our group, anatomically modern* Homo sapiens, *about 200,000 years ago."*

Given the small amount of time that has elapsed, the level of divergence between various populations is quite low, but it is not imperceptible. This means that human populations might still be distinguished by comparing a small number of different 'marker' alleles.[36,37]

The authors of the SIPRI appendix suggested that studies of non-coding regions of the human genome, particularly in genetic fingerprinting, would be of considerable importance in refining discrimination between groups. Genetic fingerprinting dates from the mid-1980s when it was discovered that there were hypervariable regions of non-coding DNA subsequently termed minisatellites.[38] There were many such minisatellites — arising from mistakes in replication — in which nucleotides were repeated in tandem. Since there is considerable variation between individuals in the numbers of repeats, and many loci of variation, characterisation of individuals became possible. The *pattern* of variation between individuals is characteristic of a particular group and differs from group to group. Evidence is accumulating that Rybeck and his co-authors were correct in their prediction. One detailed recent report concluded:[39]

> *"We have demonstrated that it is possible to identify a panel of dimorphic and microsatellite genetic markers that will allow confident EAE [ethnic-affiliation estimation] in African Americans, European Americans and Hispanic Americans....Similar sets of markers could be developed for the identification of other populations common in the United States..."*

These findings were based on the use of population-specific alleles which exhibit large frequency differentials between different population groups. Most of the alleles were "[h]ypervariable microsatellites, short tandem arrays of 2-6 bp [base pair] repeat units". The authors surveyed less than 1,000 loci for their study. As the US National Research Council's Committee on DNA Forensic Science noted in 1996:[40]

> *"One of the most promising of the newer techniques involves amplification of loci containing Short Tandem Repeats (STRs). STRs are scattered throughout the chromosomes in enormous numbers, so that there is almost unlimited potential for more loci to be discovered and validated for forensic use..."*

This suggests that many more population-specific alleles will be discovered in further research. Should it be possible to distinguish between different groups by means of a small number of marker alleles, the question then arises as to whether the different combinations of alleles might be targeted.

Gene therapy

The Swedish contribution to the background paper on new scientific and technological developments for the Fourth Review Conference of the BTWC stated:[41]

> *"...Gene therapy, still in its infancy, has been discussed in the context of gene delivery to cancer cells as well as to cells lacking a gene function. In either case, considerable challenges remain. However, a second generation of viral and non-viral vectors are already under development..."*

The important medical reasons for the development of gene therapy for cancer treatment[42] and for the correction of inborn errors of metabolism[43] are well known and can be expected to continue to generate new research in this field. It is quite probable that, despite the many current difficulties, gene therapy will be shown to have increasing practical applications in the next century. Certainly, the problems of precise location and stable expression of inserted material is likely to be the continued subject of intense research.[44] As one recent survey concluded:[45]

> *"...it seems likely that gene-based immunotherapies for some malignancies, such as neuroblastoma and melanoma, will be shown convincingly in the next few years to slow the development of further disease and to force existing tumours to regress..."*

Of course, any such success will spur on efforts to extend the technique. One possible way has been described:[46]

> *"...to introduce 'toxic' genes that will only be expressed inside the HIV-infected cell. This can be accomplished by attaching a toxic gene promoter that can only turn on expression of the toxic gene if the HIV virus resides in the cell..."*

That suggestion is obviously made for good medical reasons, but it is not difficult to see how such an approach might be misused.

Genetic weapons: Fact or fiction?

There are two obvious conclusions from this short review of the factors seen as important in the SIPRI appendix. Firstly, while genetic warfare is not, in all probability, a practical possibility today, the UK was quite correct to argue, in its 1996 background paper for the Fourth Review Conference of the BTWC, that:[47]

> *"...it cannot be ruled out that information from such genetic research could be considered for the design of weapons targeted against specific ethnic or racial groups..."*

Secondly, in view of that possibility, there is a need to keep careful watch on research in this area and to give attention to means by which malign developments can be thwarted. Whilst we should hope that genetic weapons are never developed, it would be a great mistake to assume that they never can be, and therefore that we can safely afford to ignore them as a future possibility.

CHAPTER 5

Preventing the proliferation of biological weapons

There is obviously a tension between an individual state's reasonable right to have access to weapons in order to be secure, and the danger of flooding unstable parts of the world with weaponry. It would be very hard to argue that the international community has yet found means of getting the balance right in regard to conventional weapons. All too frequently large amounts of arms are made available to fuel ongoing rivalries and conflicts. The dangers that could arise from the further spread of weapons of mass destruction make it even more important that we do not allow these to get out of control. The core argument presented here is that a great deal of future human suffering could be avoided if means can be found to prevent the further proliferation of offensive biological weapons programmes. Before reviewing the mechanisms currently available to help achieve that goal, however, there should be an awareness in technologically advanced western countries that such a goal might not be accepted without question in other parts of the world.

The ending of the east-west Cold War not only broke the bipolar framework of international security, but also left the

United States with unquestionable superiority in conventional forces at the outset of the present transitional phase of inter-state relations. This superiority is generally agreed to have come about because the US was the first country to effectively apply the revolution in information technology to warfare. US dominance in this new form of warfare was demonstrated in the 1991 Gulf War, but the history of warfare clearly indicates that other countries will not simply accept US dominance — they will respond to this new military situation. In a detailed review,[1] two analysts from the Joint Military Intelligence College in Washington DC and the US Naval Academy in Annapolis respectively, suggest that there are different types of response, one of which — a *by-passing measure* — is to conduct warfare in which the superior side's advantage cannot be relevant. An example would be a terrorist campaign targeted at the American homeland by an adversary, rather than engagement in force-on-force battles.

Counterproliferation

As the crisis over Iraq's continued restriction of UNSCOM inspections escalated in late 1997, *Jane's Defence Weekly* carried a special feature, 'Countering Weapons of Mass Destruction', in which it was argued that because of US conventional superiority, and the ease with which chemical and biological weapons could be obtained:[2]

> *"...much of the basis for US national security strategy and military planning today centres on the premise that the next time US troops deploy to a contingency in the Persian Gulf they must deal with the threat of WMD [weapons of mass destruction], and particularly chemical and biological weapons..."*

The article went on to argue that this assessment has "massive" implications and is at the root of the Clinton Administration's 1993 Counterproliferation Initiative. There are dangers if the idea of counterproliferation goes too far and pre-emptive attacks on another state, even to destroy weapons of mass destruction, are contemplated. Such attacks would not be legal under international law.[3] Yet there are obvious concerns in the United States not only about Iraq[4] but also, for example, over Iran,[5] and not just in regard to the Gulf region.[6] Indeed, in December 1997 the US Secretary of State:[7]

> *"...urged the NATO alliance...to recognize the spread of nuclear, biological and chemical weapons in the Middle East and Eurasia as its most pressing strategic priority in the post-Cold War era."*

and NATO has certainly been giving considerable attention to the problem of how to deal with WMD proliferation.[8]

It can be argued that these complex problems of differing perceptions of security and military strategy should not be important here, because what is being sought is a *total abolition* of biological weapons in just the same way as the recently agreed multilateral Chemical Weapons Convention (CWC) prescribes chemical disarmament for all parties.[9] The CWC, which entered into force in 1997 after many years of negotiation, provides for the destruction of all chemical weapons and chemical weapon production facilities, and for the regulation of the worldwide chemical industry through a complex and effective system of verification. However, despite the International Court of Justice's 1996 ruling[10] that the threat or use of nuclear weapons was generally unlawful, and that the only circumstances in which it could not definitively conclude whether the threat of use of such weapons would be lawful or unlawful was in "an extreme circumstance of self-defence, in which the very survival of a state would be at stake", nuclear weapons will not be abolished quickly. The arguments about the meaning of the International Court's ruling are complex but, on balance, whilst the judgement may have strictly confined the legality of the possession or use of such weapons, it did not state that they were definitely illegal in all circumstances. Moreover, states still appear to be willing to contemplate use of nuclear weapons.[11,12]

The development of nuclear weapons and their entrenchment in military systems has been underway for only fifty years. We can take steps now to make it less likely that they are ever used again, but it seems probable that removing nuclear weapons altogether is a task that will take decades. The key point here is that the current differences over the imbalance in the distribution of *nuclear* weapons should not prevent us doing whatever we can to abolish *biological* weapons. Biological weapons are presently less entrenched in military systems and should therefore be easier to control. If we wait until they are further entrenched, abolition will be much more difficult to achieve. Furthermore, the proliferation of biological weapons of mass destruction is hardly likely to make the process of nuclear disarmament any easier,[13,14,15] and nuclear disarmament is clearly imperative for survival of the species in the longer term.[16] That is not to argue that we can, therefore, ignore the possibility of different perceptions of the utility of biological weapons in different parts of the world. Indeed, the existence of these differing perceptions about the utility of weapons of mass destruction means that it is necessary to analyse such differences more carefully, in order to design appropriate policies that will lead to the total prohibition of biological weapons.

The motivations which lead a state to seek to acquire biological weapons are likely to be complex,[17] and all have to be taken into account in framing a policy to prevent proliferation. As Michael Moodie has noted, we are not just dealing with a simple matter of trying to prevent the proliferation of weapons systems.[18] Thinking only in terms of weapons and threats can lead to narrow analyses of short-term military options[19] when all such options appear to have substantial drawbacks.[20] As Moodie points out, modern biotechnology brings major economic benefits, as well as improving capabilities for producing offensive biological weapons, and so:

"...denying technology to a potential recipient will be neither possible nor justifiable in the light of the commercial utility of the technology..."

Thus he argues that our problem lies not just in controlling the diffusion of technology, and perhaps not even in the technology itself, but in influencing the choices of those to whom technology is available. In short, how do we ensure that dual-use technology is used for benign ends and not in offensive biological weapons programmes?

The international norm that biological weapons are unacceptable

Any system designed to ensure that dual-use technology is used for benign ends and not in offensive biological weapons programmes must necessarily be centred on the norm embodied in the 1925 Geneva Protocol and the 1972 Biological and Toxin Weapons Convention (BTWC), which categorise biological weapons as unacceptable to the international community.[21] Only when such weapons are effectively subject to a global prohibition regime[22] can we ensure that offensive biological weapons programmes are a most unlikely possibility. Our problem today is that for biological weapons (which are the easiest of the weapons of mass destruction to procure), the control system is by far the weakest.[23] Table 5.1 demonstrates clearly how much needs to be done to strengthen this regime. The poverty of the capabilities embodied in the BTWC as compared to the CWC is particularly noteworthy.

When the Cold War ended there was a brief period when it appeared that the need for arms control agreements was also at an end. However, it soon became clear that this was a misunderstanding based on the domination of arms control concepts by a very restricted notion of the scope of the agreements that had been evolved by the international community over time,

Table 5.1: Rule of law attributes of arms control treaties*

Treaty	Foreswear actions	Take actions	Refer disputes	Establish Organization	Verify	Provide for sanctions	Require national measures
Geneva Protocol of 1925	✔						
Limited Test Ban Treaty of 1963	✔						
Biological Weapons Convention of 1972	✔	✔	✔				
Nuclear Non-Proliferation Safeguards Agreement of 1972	✔	✔	✔	✔	✔	✔	
Intermediate Range Nuclear Forces Agreement of 1972	✔	✔		✔	✔		
Strategic Arms Reduction Treaty of 1991	✔	✔		✔	✔		
Chemical Weapons Convention of 1993	✔	✔	✔	✔	✔	✔	✔

*From[24]

as different challenges were met in different historical periods.[25] As Tanzman has argued:[26]

> "...the end of the Cold War marks a shift away from reliance on military might towards an international commitment to

control weapons of mass destruction through the 'rule of law'..."

The endpoint of the process we may be engaged in was described last year by Ambassador Leonard, the US negotiator of the original BTWC:[27]

"During the long, slow transition to a new system of international relations, the global and regional arms control treaties of the past 40 years will be complemented by additional treaty regimes covering the full range of conventional weapons..."

He continued:

"...Together, these treaties will provide a framework of norms, obligations, procedures, rules and interactions that will foster political advances..."

The international system will eventually be transformed:

"...These treaties will bring with them a matrix of verification procedures so penetrating, so ubiquitous and so intrusive as to be unimaginable today. Total transparency in military matters will be the norm that is steadily and inexorably approached. Military secrecy will be seen, increasingly, as an unhealthy remnant of a previous era in which national security was protected by the balance of power."

An alternative view sees a continuation of a security system based on balances of power amongst an increasing multiplicity of states armed with various weapons of mass destruction. The problem with a continuing balance of power system in the modern world is that the traditional security dilemma will be increasingly exacerbated by the presence of weapons of mass destruction. Traditionally, the security dilemma has implied that the more a state armed in order to improve its security, the more surrounding states were likely to feel insecure and to arm in response. This would then set up a positive feedback process of endless armament. The presence of weapons of mass destruction compounds the problem because they may severely increase the pressures towards using such weapons first before the other parties to a conflict use them on you. Clearly this could greatly increase instability in conflict-prone regions. Ambassador Leonard's prescription for the future implies a negative feedback process being set in motion in which less and less weaponry is required. The increased transparency provides assurance of security for all, and leads to a much more stable and less conflict-prone world system. If we are to set out on the road Ambassador Leonard prescribes, our main task today is to complete the process of strengthening the BTWC.

Strengthening the Biological and Toxin Weapons Convention

As noted in Chapter 3, at the third Five Year Review Conference of the Convention in 1991, the States Parties decided to confirm and develop the efforts they had initiated in 1986 to increase transparency through 'Confidence Building Measures' in the form of voluntary annual data exchanges. In the aftermath of the 1991 Gulf War they also decided to set up a process — VEREX — by which a scientific analysis would be made of the possibility of verifying the Convention. The positive final report of the VEREX group[28] was considered at a Special Conference of States Parties in 1994, and this mandated an Ad Hoc Group of government experts to continue the process.[29] The mandate given to the Ad Hoc Group in 1994 is shown in Table 5.2.

Whilst the relatively weak possibility of investigation of alleged use under the BTWC through Convention Article VI had been considerably reinforced by Security Council Resolution 620 of 1988[31] and General Assembly Resolution 45/57/C (on guidelines and procedures), it is important to note that the Ad Hoc Group

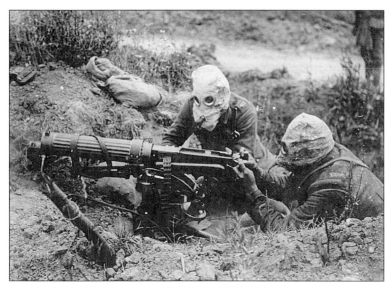

Figure i: Chemical weapons were used on the battlefields in the First World War. Protective clothing being worn at the Battle of the Somme.

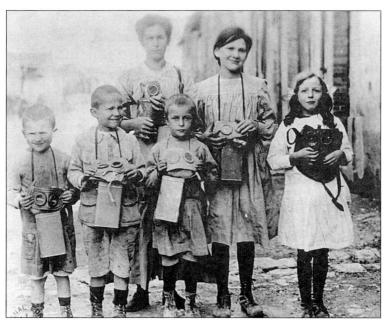

Figure ii: Civil defence preparations in France. The deployment of chemical weapons in the First World War led to the 1925 Geneva Convention banning the use of chemical and biological weapons.

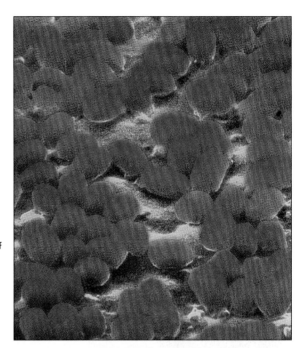

Figure iii: Coloured scanning electron micrograph (SEM) of *Bacillus anthracis* spores. 100 kg of anthrax spores spread effectively over a city in the right conditions might kill 1 to 3 million people.

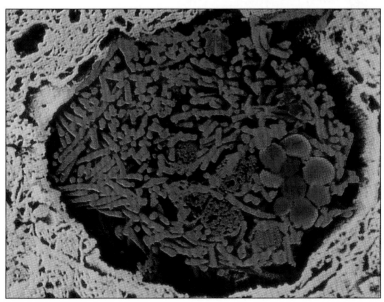

Figure iv: *Bacillus anthracis* (the causative bacterium of anthrax), in a capillary of a lung. Spongy tissues surrounding the capillary are lung alveoli. The rod-shaped Gram positive bacteria are highly pathogenic. Pulmonary anthrax is fatal in most cases.

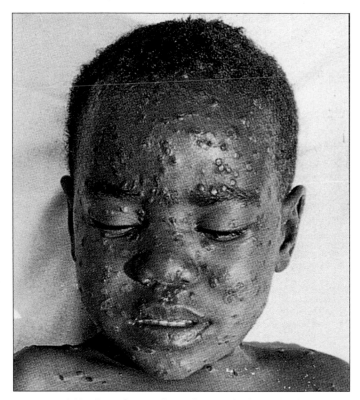

Figure v: A child suffering from smallpox infection. The disease has been eradicated by the WHO's vaccination programme. Evidence suggests, however, that smallpox may be one of the biological agents being investigated in the former Soviet Union for its potential weapons use.

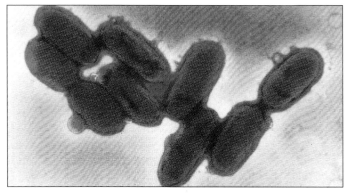

Figure vi: *Yersinia pestis*. Coloured transmission electron micrograph of a cluster of the bacterium *Yersinia pestis*, cause of bubonic plague. Infection is rapid, causing swollen lymph nodes, and leading to septicaemia and pulmonary infection.

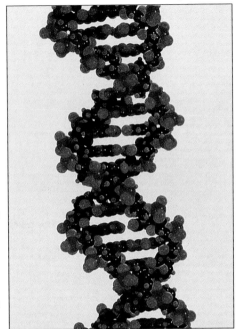

Figure vii: Model representation of DNA (deoxyribonucleic acid) the genetic material of most living organisms. The mapping of the human genetic code will bring many benefits to medical science and the early detection and prevention of disease. Such knowledge, however, could also be used to enhance known pathogens, for example, to create antibiotic resistant biological strains of bacteria.

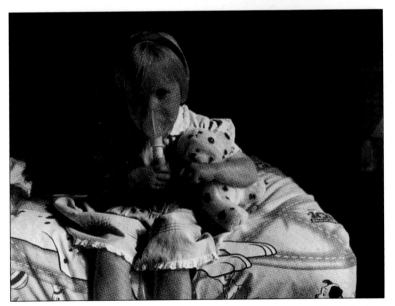

Figure viii: Alexandra Preston, a 4 year old sufferer of cystic fibrosis. Cystic fibrosis is one of the many genetic disorders that could benefit from advances in the understanding of human genetics.

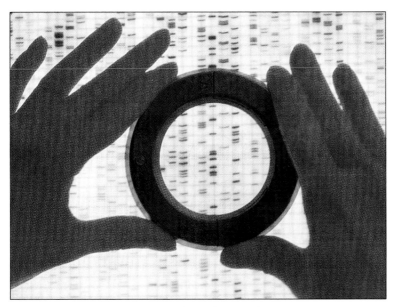

Figure ix: Circular computer 'scanner' used to read sections of DNA sequencing autoradiographs for subsequent computer analysis, part of the human genome project studies at CalTech, USA — one of the many laboratories worldwide engaged in various aspects of genome research.

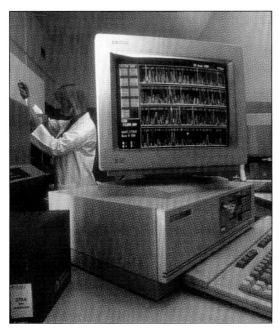

Figure x: Mapping the human genome: computer equipment used at CEPH, St Louis Hospital, France to analyse the DNA sequence of the HL-A system, a gene cluster located in chromosome 6 in humans. The HL-A gene complex has been implicated in many aspects of immunology.

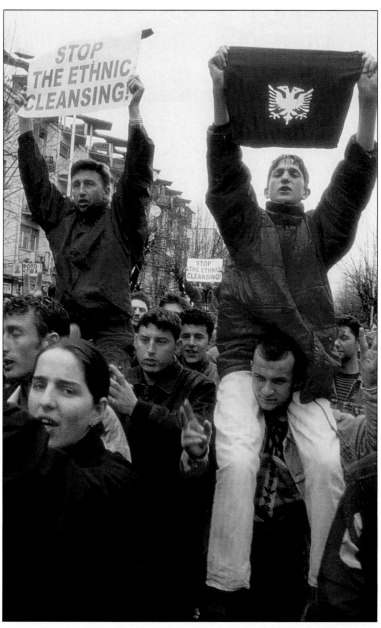

Figure xi: The closing decades of the 20th century have borne witness to many atrocities against ethnic populations. Kosovo crisis: 9th March 1998, ethnic Albanians demonstrate against Serbian aggression.

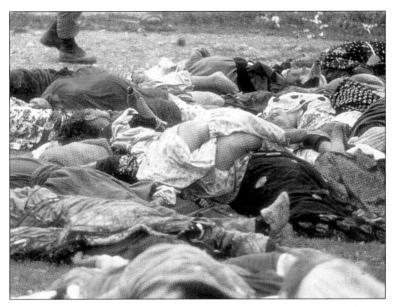

Figure xii: Chemical weapons attack on the Kurdish population in Halabja by Iraqi forces in 1988.

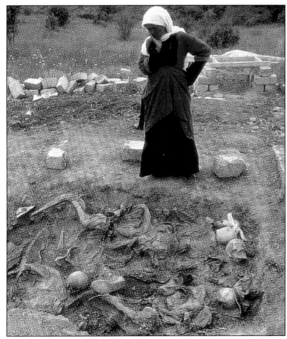

Figure xiii: A widow examines a mass grave in Kurdistan, 1992.

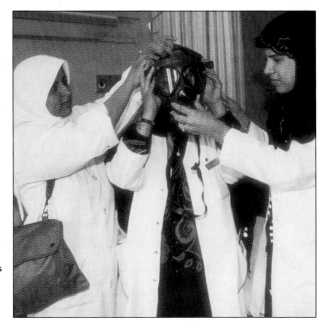

Figure xiv: Doctors in the frontline: Kuwaiti nurses help a doctor put on a gas mask during the Gulf War.

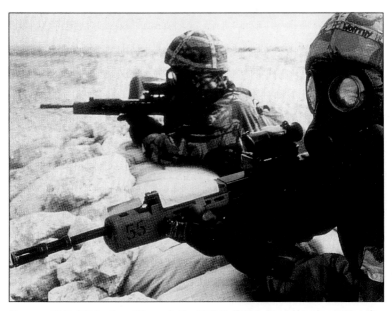

Figure xv: United States Armed Forces in the 1991 Gulf War. Troops wearing NBC outfits carry out a training exercise. The threat of chemical and biological attack was taken very seriously by coalition forces.

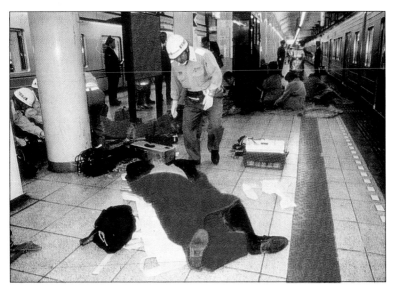

Figure xvi: The aftermath of the Tokyo sarin nerve gas attack in 1995.

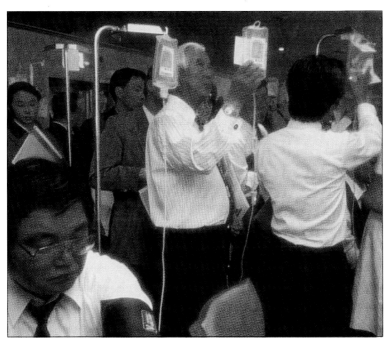

Figure xvii: Twelve people were killed and over 5,000 injured in the Tokyo sarin nerve gas attack by the Aum Shinrikyo sect.

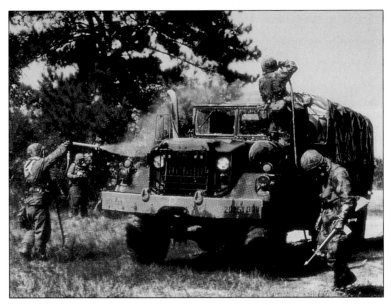

Figure xviii: Joint US and UK military exercise, Fort Mclellan, Alabama (1998). Preparing for chemical and biological attack.

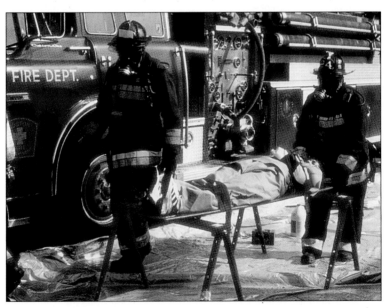

Figure xix: Civil defence preparations, Boston. Emergency services simulate a response to chemical or biological attack.

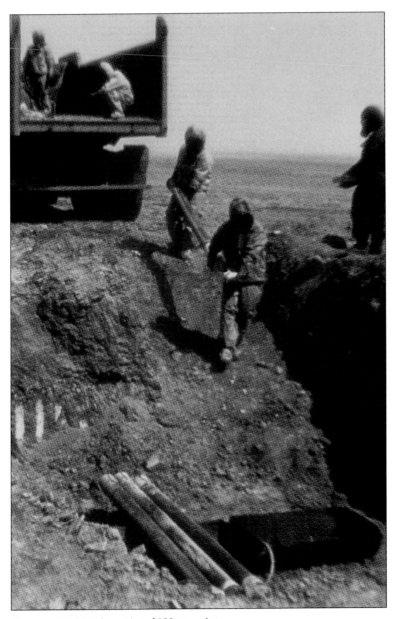

Figure xx: UNSCOM destruction of 122mm rockets.

Since 1991 UNSCOM has directed and supervised the destruction or rendering harmelss of several identified facilities and large quantities of equipment for the production of chemical and biological weapons as well as proscribed long-range missiles.

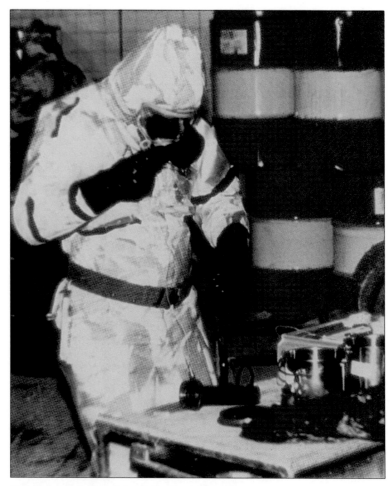

Figure xxi: Examination of chemical weapon precursors.

UNSCOM personnel carry out on-site inspections of Iraq's biological, chemical and missile capabilities in order to monitor and verify Iraq's compliance with its unconditional obligation not to use, retain, process, develop, construct or otherwise acquire weapons of mass destruction.

Table 5.2: Mandate given to the new Ad Hoc Group by the 1994 Special Conference*

"The Conference also recognized that the complex nature of the issues pertaining to the strengthening of the Biological Weapons Convention underlined the need for a gradual approach towards the establishment of a coherent regime to enhance the effectivenes of and improve compliance with the Convention. **This regime would include,** *inter alia,* **potential verification measures, as well as agreed procedures and mechanisms for their efficient implementation and measures for the investigation of alleged use.**

...The objective of this Ad Hoc Group shall be to consider appropriate measures, including possible verification measures, and draft proposals to strengthen the Convention, to be included, as appropriate, in a legally binding instrument, to be submitted for the consideration of the States Parties. In this context, the Ad Hoc Group shall, *inter alia* consider:

- Definitions of terms and objective criteria...

- The incorporation of existing and further enhanced confidence building and transparency measures...

- A system of measures to promote compliance with the Convention, including, as appropriate, measures identified, examined and evaluated in the VEREX Report...

- Specific measures designed to ensure effective and full implementation of Article X...

Measures should be formulated and implemented in a manner designed to protect sensitive commercial proprietary information and legitimate national security needs.

Measures shall be formulated and implemented in a manner designed to avoid any negative impact on scientific research, international cooperation and industrial development."

*From[30]

mandate does include "measures for the investigation of alleged use" in the proposed regime. Also included for consideration are Confidence Building Measures and co-operation under Article X of the Convention (see Table 6.1). Central to the aim of strengthening the BTWC is the "system of measures to promote compliance with the Convention". Definitions of terms and objective criteria are clearly necessary where they are relevant to implementation of the specific measures agreed.

The new Ad Hoc Group had a first procedural meeting in January 1995 and a further series of meetings in Geneva during 1995 and 1996. At that stage, after the fifth meeting, the group reported to the Fourth Review Conference of the BTWC in late 1996. The Group was asked to negotiate the text of a Verification Protocol and to finish its work before the Fifth Review Conference in 2001.

The Ad Hoc Group went on to meet for several sessions in 1997. At the seventh session of the Ad Hoc Group, the Chairman, Ambassador Tibor Tóth, presented a "Rolling Text of a Protocol to the Convention" based on the progress which had been made up to the end of the sixth session. It is this text which is now being developed by the Ad Hoc Group. At the end of the eighth session in September/October 1997 it contained 23 Articles, eight Annexes and five Appendices. Extracts from Annex A.II Lists and Criteria (Agents and Toxins) can be found in Appendix 3.[32] The pace of negotiations is increasing, with eleven weeks of negotiations scheduled for 1998. However, few professional scientists appeared even to be aware of the negotiations, even though the developing text was available on the Internet.[33]

Ambassador Tóth suggested, in a review in late 1997, that four clusters of issues needed to be given priority:[34]

> "...One cluster concerns on-site visits and investigations and another what kind of declarations there should be. A further set of issues relates to definitions, lists and criteria and a fourth set addressing Article X (scientific and technical cooperation) and Article III (non-transfer measures)..."

Though there are other issues that will need resolving, these four seem to encapsulate the key difficulties that will have to be dealt with in the coming final stages of the negotiations.

Powerful industrial interests, concerned about the potential loss of Confidential Business Information (CBI), favour what is known as a two-pillar verification regime in which declarations are backed up by only one form of on-site measure — challenge *investigations* of non-compliance concerns.[35] Others view this approach as inadequate and argue that there should be two forms of on-site measures — non-challenge *visits* to declared sites as well as challenge investigations of any site. Their contrary argument is based on the view that there will not be large numbers of declared sites and routine visits as in the Chemical Weapons Convention, but that it is necessary to have visits, in addition to challenge investigations, in order to be able to check, for example, the consistency of declarations. Linked to this issue is the lack of any organisation to maintain the BTWC between review conferences. Clearly, an organisation to operate the Verification Protocol will be a necessity, but it seems unlikely that it will be of the same scale and cost as the CWC organisation.

In regard to differences over definitions, lists and so on, Ambassador Tóth suggested that these differences can be resolved pragmatically by confining any necessary definitions to the *Protocol*. This would avoid any misunderstanding which might arise if definitions were built into the *Convention* itself. Clearly, if what was intended to be an illustrative listing of what could be covered by Article I of the Convention was taken to be a definitive list of what was actually covered, then there would be scope for many problems to arise. Putting the definitions and lists into the Protocol makes it quite clear that these are aids to the present implementation of the Convention and in no way limit the General Purpose Criterion embedded in Article I of the Convention.

There is unlikely to be a simple resolution to the final set of issues concerning Article X and Article III. It has to be understood that many developing countries among the 140 States Parties to the BTWC see the Convention as a bargain in which their support for arms control brings economic benefits through scientific and technological co-operation under Article X. In this view, export controls — particularly co-ordinated export controls by advanced industrial countries — under Article III of the Convention will have to be reconsidered as the Protocol is developed. Such differences over export controls have caused problems at BTWC

Review Conferences in the past,[36] and in the final stages of the negotiation of the CWC.[37]

This point was made by the Non-Aligned Movement in a statement in March 1998. Whilst stressing their support for completion of negotiations according to the Ad Hoc Group's mandate, this stated that they:[38]

> *"...wish to stress that the mandate under which the Ad-Hoc Group is carrying out this work needs to be implemented fully. In this regard they express their concerns at attempts to reduce the scope and importance of issues related to Article X of the Convention, which may be prejudicial to the declared objective of intensification of the work of the Ad-Hoc Group..."*

It would seem important that technologically advanced states take notice of this warning because the support of the Non-Aligned Movement will be crucial in achieving a successful outcome to the negotiations. On the other hand, a very positive move was made in early 1998 when the United States announced its firm supportive position regarding completion of substantive negotiation of the Verification Protocol by the end of 1998.[39] This was followed by a strong statement from the European Union.[40] The position adopted by the United States was important because it could have been argued that strengthening the Convention was low down on its list of arms control priorities, which was still dominated by bilateral nuclear issues,[41] and that this was reflected in the difficulties it had in agreeing a position in regard to the BTWC negotiations.

Summarising the situation in early 1998, one authoritative commentator concluded:[42]

> *"The AHG [Ad Hoc Group] has made excellent progress. What is needed is the political momentum to complete the negotiations. The elements of the integrated compliance regime and the organization are largely already there in the rolling text for the Protocol and the issues that yet have to be*

> *elaborated are those related primarily to [national] implementation (Article IV), international cooperation (Article X) and non-transfer (Article III)..."*

In short, the technical discussions are proceeding well, but there is a need for political will to complement that progress and push the negotiations to a close. That political will would in turn be greatly enhanced by more widespread specialist and popular knowledge of the issue. The question of what might be done to enhance political will is considered in the next chapter. First, it should be noted that while reinforcement of the norm of non-use is the essential, *central* component of a system of restraint on offensive biological weapons programmes, and use of such weapons, several other elements are also required.

The web of deterrence

Given the complexities of the mechanisms and motivations that may underlie acquisition and use of biological weapons, it is not surprising that careful analyses[43,44,45] of what needs to be done to prevent such dangers suggest some form of what has been called[46] a "web of deterrence" (Table 5.3). The aim of such a set of integrated policies is to convince a potential proliferator that a CBW (chemical and biological warfare) capability is not worthwhile.

Table 5.3: Elements of the web of deterrence*

- Comprehensive, verifiable, and global CB arms control to create a risk of detection and a climate of political unacceptability for CB weapons;

- Broad export monitoring and controls to make it difficult and expensive for a proliferator to obtain necessary materials;

- Effective CB defensive and protective measures to reduce the military utility of CB weapons; and

- A range of determined and effective national and international responses to CB acquisition and/or use.

*From[47]

Table 5.4: Types of use of biological weapons*

1. Terrorist or Individual use

Scale of attack	Nature of aggressor		
	Individual	Subnational Group	State Party
Point source	Criminal acts	Covert terrorist or national liberation attack Assassination	—
Medium scale	Criminal acts	Terrorist attack	—
Large scale	Criminal acts (not normally possible)	—	—

2. Covert Use

Scale of attack	Nature of aggressor		
	Individual	Subnational Group	State Party
Point source	Criminal acts	Covert terrorist or national liberation attack Assassination	National covert operations Assassination
Medium scale	—	—	—
Large scale	—	—	—

3. Military Use

Scale of attack	Nature of aggressor		
	Individual	Subnational Group	State Party
Point source	—	—	—
Medium scale	—	National liberation military use	Military tactical use
Large scale	—	National liberation military use	Military tactical and strategic use

*From[49]

In regard to the first element of the web, comprehensive arms control, it will be recalled (Tables 2.7 and 2.8) that Wheelis[48] proposed a three-point typology of biological warfare involving the nature of the aggressor, the scale of attack and the identity of the target. He then produced a nine-cell matrix of possible types of biological warfare by combining the nature of the aggressor with the scale of attack. Obviously, each of the possible types of biological warfare could be targeted against humans, animals or plants. What is of particular interest here is that Wheelis went on to suggest that it was possible to envisage three types of *use* of biological weapons (Table 5.4) and three strategies of deterrence or detection appropriate to each category of use (Table 5.5).

Table 5.5: Strategies for deterring or detecting types of biological warfare*

To deter or detect terrorist or criminal use

1. Increased encouragement of States Parties to enact and enforce strong legislation implementing Article IV.

To deter or detect covert use

2. Measures allowing on-site investigation of suspicious outbreaks of infectious disease or intoxination, and of allegations of use.

3. Measures enhancing the epidemiological and disease control capabilities of States Parties.

To deter or detect military programs

4. Measures allowing on-site inspection of munitions production facilities and/or deployed and stockpiled munitions to detect bioweapon delivery devices.

5. Measures allowing on-site inspection of microbial growth facilities that could be diverted to BW agent production.

*From[50]

In regard to military programmes (Table 5.5, points 4 and 5), as Wheelis notes, little attention has been paid in the open literature to dealing with actual weaponry (measures under point 4). What is clear, however, from the continuing problems with

Iraq,[51] is the enormous difficulty and expense of mounting such an operation against a single state. The argument for strengthening the multilateral BTWC, to deter any such programme in the future and to provide legitimate means of investigating possible non-compliance (measures under point 5), is therefore greatly reinforced.

Wheelis' analysis very clearly draws attention to two other aspects of the BTWC: the requirement under Article IV to enact appropriate national legislation (Table 5.5, point 1); and measures to deter or detect covert use (Table 5.5, points 2 and 3). Measures to allow on-site investigations of alleged use, as we have seen (Table 5.2), are already part of the mandate of the current Ad Hoc Group. In regard to the measure under point 3 of Table 5.5 — enhancing the epidemiological and disease control capabilities of States Parties — Wheelis suggests:

> *"Such measures, which might include epidemiological and medical training, enhanced electronic linkages, provision of diagnostic reagents and medications, expanded clinical facilities, and expansion of databases on infectious diseases are important ways of implementing Article X..."*

He adds that the provision of such capabilities around the world may, in the longer term, be the best way of deterring covert use of biological weapons.

The question of covert use arose for the States Parties to the BTWC in 1997 when Cuba accused the United States of releasing plant-destroying insects over its agricultural land[52] and asked Russia to raise the issue under Article V of the Convention.[53] Cuba's case does not appear to have been substantiated. However, considerable expertise is available for the investigation of allegations of use from professionals who have to investigate natural outbreaks of disease,[54] and it seems likely that the Ad Hoc Group will have the technical capability to produce a satisfactory outcome for this part of their mandate. Nevertheless, there are considerable political sensitivities in Russia and in member countries of the Non-Aligned Movement to investigations of disease outbreaks that will need to be overcome.[55]

At the time the BTWC was negotiated, a few countries, including the UK,[56] enacted national measures of the kind required by Article IV but, despite exhortation by successive Five Year Review Conferences, the number of countries with national legislation remains small.[57] However, there has been an obvious increase in concern about the possible use of biological weapons by terrorists[58,59,60] and, in order to cope with this potential threat, substantial analysis[61] and allocation of resources[62,63] are urgently required. Amongst the set of responses to terrorism is the enactment of national legislation (Table 5.5, measures under point 1). It is clear from the experience of the United States that this legislation will have to be complex and will necessarily extend regulation of many civil biotechnology activities substantially. Over the last decade the US Congress has developed a quite comprehensive legal framework to prevent the illegal use of toxins and infectious biological agents[64], including stricter monitoring on location and transfer of hazardous biological agents.

The second element in the suggested web of deterrence (Table 5.3) is a set of broad export controls designed to make it difficult for a proliferator to obtain the materials needed to produce biological weapons. Such controls are certainly required under Article III of the BTWC, and their importance is underlined by the way Iraq set about procuring what was needed for its offensive biological weapons programme. Some 30 countries now co-ordinate their export controls through the Australia Group,[65] which was formed in 1984 following use of chemical weapons in the Iran-Iraq War.[66] The Australia Group controls (Table 5.6) have been a cause of considerable resentment amongst the Non-Aligned Movement.[67]

The Non-Aligned countries argue that with a Verification Protocol package such controls will no longer be necessary. Western states, however, feel that these controls have been useful and do not appear willing to relinquish them. The tension identified by Ambassador Tóth[69] between the requirements of

Table 5.6: Australia Group controls in relation to biological weapons proliferation*

- Core list of agents including 20 viruses, 13 bacteria, four rickettsiae, 10 toxins, and genetically modified micro-organisms derived from agents on the core list.

- *Dual-use biological equipment* particularly well-suited for production or testing of biological weapons such as stainless steel fermentation tanks, freeze-drying equipment and aerosol inhalation chambers.

- An informal 'warning list' to industry of dual-use materials and equipment.

*From[68]

Articles III (non-transfer measures) and X (scientific and technical cooperation) of the BTWC will not be easily resolved.

The third element of the web of deterrence is not as directly related to the BTWC. Effective chemical and biological defensive and protective measures can obviously reduce the attractiveness of such weapons. Biological defence programmes,[70,71] given the possible misperception that they may mask offensive aspects, have in the past been subject to considerable criticism.[72,73] Nevertheless, defensive programmes are necessary and some elements of secrecy seem sensible — for example, in relation to key vulnerabilities. What should be required is the maximum possible openness and transparency in order to maintain democratic control and public support.

The deficiencies in detection capabilities encountered by coalition forces during the 1991 Gulf War triggered greatly increased research and development,[74] for example on detection systems.[75] There is obviously potential for improving force protection, and detection and identification of biological agents of concern.[76,77] Similarly, there are opportunities for building on the considerable knowledge of medical countermeasures that may be taken against the use of biological weapons that we already have.[78]

Of course, all elements of a web of deterrence are enhanced to the extent that the international community gains knowledge of the activities of potential proliferators. To encourage people to expose such activity it is necessary to reinforce the norm which stigmatises biological weapons as unacceptable. Scientific specialists in technologically advanced countries would appear to have particular responsibilities in regard to the monitoring of developments in their areas of expertise. For example, specialists would surely be the first to know if genetic weapons were becoming a practical possibility. They would therefore appear to have a special responsibility, first to be aware that this problem might arise and then to be in a position to help prevent it happening through taking action individually, and also through their professional associations.

Finally, when considering the presently available means of preventing the proliferation of biological weapons it is necessary to note sanctions. It is clear that without a verifiable multilateral convention it is proving ever more difficult to maintain the consensus for keeping pressure on Iraq to demonstrate finally and unequivocally that it has no biological weapons.[79] This is despite widespread agreement that the international community should have reacted very strongly to Iraqi use of chemical weapons — particularly against civilians at Halabja — in the 1980s. The US bombing of the pharmaceutical factory in Sudan in August 1998 illustrates the difficulties of appropriate sanctions and clear responses to allegations of biological weapons development. Much additional thought is required on how a range of determined and effective responses to violations of the norm (Table 5.3) are to be constructed and used.[80]

Chapter 6

Summary: The web of deterrence

New biological weapons

Biological warfare has been a persistent threat to world health and security. Historical evidence summarised in this report has shown that although there has been a strong prohibition against the use of biological weapons and toxins, offensive research has continued, and many nation states have extensive biological warfare programmes. Nations suspected by the Office of Technology Assessment, and at the US Senate hearings in 1995, of having offensive biological weapons programmes included Iran, Iraq, Libya, Syria, North Korea, Taiwan, Israel, Egypt, Vietnam, Laos, Cuba, Bulgaria, India, South Korea, South Africa, China and Russia. As we reach the end of the millennium it is important that we take account of the continuing threat that these weapons are posing to humanity. As one military commentator has argued:[1]

> "Although many people believe that biological warfare in the twentieth century has been a rare phenomenon, biological warfare (BW) and fear of BW have affected our wars, our peace, our treaties and our research throughout this century..."

This report has focused on the possibility that new advances in our understanding of the human genome could be used to enhance biological warfare programmes. The Human Genome Project is likely to come to fruition, as planned, in the early years of the next century and will probably be seen as crystallising our knowledge of modern biology. It will then underpin the further massive expansion of biotechnology and molecular medicine that will drive pivotal industries in the first half of the next century. So while our immediate concern must be to strengthen the Biological and Toxin Weapons Convention and to take reasonable precautions against possible near-term use of biological weapons, we must also look carefully at means by which effective regulation of biological weapons may be further enhanced over a much longer time-scale. Knowledge derived from these developments could be used to enhance the lethality of biological organisms dangerous to human health, or could even be applied in weapons to target particular ethnic groups. This latter potential is particularly worrying given the historical prevalence of genocide and ethnic conflict.

Advances in genetic engineering, made possible by the mapping of the human genome, while undoubtedly beneficial to the human race, create frightening new possibilities for BW development — such possibilities make preventive arms regulation and the strengthening of the BTWC paramount. The scientific community and medical profession need to be aware of the potential misuse of this new technology, and strengthen the 'web of deterrence' against BW and genetic weapons. This web of deterrence includes strengthening ethical codes, monitoring the research of fellow scientists to prevent the malign use of such knowledge, and strengthening civil defence and emergency response preparations in the event of actual misuse. At present there is no clear evidence that any nation state or terrorist organisation has embarked on a substantial BW programme involving genetically engineered weapons. This therefore makes prohibition a priority. If we wait until they are firmly entrenched in military regimes, abolition will be much more difficult to achieve. Our present priority should be to strengthen the Biological and Toxin Weapons Convention.

The Biological and Toxin Weapons Convention Verification Protocol

The outline of what is needed currently to strengthen the BTWC is clear.[2] All the necessary elements can be seen in the Rolling Text of the Protocol (Table 6.1). The question is whether this technical progress can be complemented by the generation of sufficient political will to see the negotiations through to early completion.

The difficulties lying ahead, which could seriously disrupt negotiation of the BTWC Verification Protocol, have been well illustrated by the problems involved in maintaining a consensus amongst permanent members of the Security Council over what to do about Iraq's offensive biological weapons programme. The crisis of late 1997-early 1998 was eventually defused by the UN Secretary General reaching an agreement in Iraq.[4] However, the new mechanism requested by Iraq, of a technical evaluation meeting (TEM) between experts, has so far produced no change in UNSCOM's position. The group of 18 experts from 15 countries who met Iraqi officials for a week in March 1998 stated:[5]

> "...No additional confidence in the veracity and expanse of the FFCD [Iraq's full, final and complete declaration] was derived from the TEM. Iraq did not provide any new technical information of substance to support its FFCD."

The subsequent full UNSCOM report to the Security Council concluded:[6]

> "...Iraq's claim, uttered repeatedly and sometimes stridently during the period under review — to the effect that it is now absolutely free of any prohibited weapons and the equipment used to make them...has not been able to be verified..."

91

Table 6.1: A Verification Protocol for the BTWC*

Compliance Monitoring

    a.   Mandatory Declarations of those facilities and activities of most relevance to the Convention.

    b.   Non-Challenge Visits, both focused and random, to declared facilities.

    c.   Compliance Concern Investigations, both facility and field.

Article III Measures (Non-Transfer)

    a.   Guidelines for transfer of biological agents, toxins and equipment.

    b.   Requirement for annual declarations by States Parties.

    c.   Provisions for investigations of concerns that a transfer has occurred in breach of Article III of the Convention.

Article IV Measures (National Implementation)

    a.   Requirements for States Parties to enact penal legislation to implement the prohibition of any activity prohibited under the Convention.

    b.   Requirement for States Parties to set up a National Authority to implement the Protocol.

    c.   Requirements for States Parties to report to the BTWC Organization on the national laws, regulations, administrative and other national measures that it has taken to implement Article IV of the Convention.

Article X Measures (Cooperation for Peaceful Purposes)

    a.   Measures to facilitate the harmonisation of national, regional and international safety rules for pathogens involving both the collection of data and the inspection of facilities.

    b.   Measures to assist countries to adopt internationally harmonised standards for GMP [Good Manufacturing Practice] of pharmaceutical products and to establish national inspectorates to carry out regular inspections of pharmaceutical manufacturers.

*From[3]

In short, as the final negotiation phase of the BTWC Verification Protocol got underway, the permanent members of the Security Council seemed likely to have to confront again the problem over which they had so recently been completely divided.[7] The chances of agreeing an effective strengthening of the BTWC — if Iraq is not forced to show that it has given up its offensive biological programme — are surely much reduced, and the likelihood of achieving a consensus over how to enforce Iraqi compliance remains remote.

It has to be said, in view of this and other obvious possible difficulties involved in agreeing a Verification Protocol for the BTWC, that the present opportunity to strengthen the Convention could be lost. It is particularly obvious that there is little understanding of what is at stake, either amongst scientific specialists or the general public. The kind of media attention and groundswell of support that underpinned the recent agreement to ban anti-personnel landmines in the Ottawa process is going to be difficult to generate in the time, to 2001, which realistically is available for agreeing the Verification Protocol. This does not mean that an agreement to strengthen the Convention cannot be achieved, or that other means of helping to prevent the proliferation and possible use of biological weapons are pre-empted.

North-South co-operation in the fight against disease

One of the really serious divisions between the States Parties to the BTWC, that between the advanced industrial states and the less technologically developed states over Article X co-operation, does seem to be more susceptible to a favourable outcome if viewed in a wider context. Though some states from the South are primarily concerned about restrictions on industrial development, it is not as if they can be treated as a single bloc. These states have varying interests and many would support the BTWC if there was a reasonable gain in terms of dealing with basic needs.[8] Modern biotechnology and medicine have important roles to play in dealing with such problems if they are properly applied.[9] Whilst the problems of disease in the developing world, for example, are widely known,[10] it is less well understood in the developed world that infectious diseases remain a potential problem for us,[11] particularly as drug resistance increases,[12] and we encounter new diseases.[13] It is therefore vital, both for the developed and developing worlds, to have a high degree of disease surveillance so that new dangers can be identified and dealt with rapidly. Unfortunately there is widespread concern amongst specialists about the present state of disease surveillance,[14] and important issues that need to be resolved by the World Health Organization in the ongoing revision of its system of epidemic control.[15]

It has been pointed out (see Chapter 5) that there is a potential synergy here between efforts to strengthen the BTWC and those to improve the world's system of natural disease monitoring. The better the international civil system of disease monitoring, the less likely the deliberate use of disease agents will go undetected. This idea has been considerably elaborated by concerned scientists[16,17] and a prototype non-governmental reporting system (ProMED-mail) was put on the Internet by the Federation of American Scientists in 1994.[18] There has also been much work on a wider-ranging system for countering emerging diseases, linked to the strengthening of the BTWC.[19] Whatever emerges under the Article X co-operation aspect of the strengthening of the Convention can therefore be seen as part of this broader international effort to deal with the ever-present threat of pathogens.

Co-operation to counter terrorism

In addition to state-sponsored programmes (which may put pressure on the scientific and medical communities to participate in biological weapons research), contemporary concerns have also focused on the potential use of biological weapons by terrorist organisations or cults.

Some recent examples of attempts to obtain or develop biological weapons have proven that this is more than just a theoretical possibility.

• The Aum Shinrikyo cult in Japan were responsible for a Sarin attack on the Tokyo subway in 1995 which killed a dozen people and injured 5000. In 1992 members of the cult had travelled to Zaire to help victims of the Ebola outbreak, but a report by the US Senate's Permanent Subcommittee on Investigations concluded that the cult had probably intended to obtain virus samples for biological attacks.[20] Prominent cult members included a cardiovascular surgeon and several graduate scientists.[21]

- In May 1995 Larry Harris, a laboratory technician in Ohio, ordered the bacterium that causes bubonic plague, and was mailed three vials of *Yersinia pestis*. To obtain these bacteria, Harris only needed a credit card and a false letterhead. Harris later claimed that he wanted to conduct research to combat Iraqi rats carrying 'supergerms' and he was found to be a member of a white supremacist organisation.[22]

In addition, 'recipes' for making biological weapons are freely available on the Internet. We must create additional safeguards to prevent rogue individuals from using the tools of biotechnology for malign purposes — and scientists must monitor colleagues who may be passing on information or giving assistance to bioterrorist research. This task is equal in importance to that of preventing the national proliferation of biological weapons in state-sponsored programmes. It is clear that such terrorism cannot be completely eliminated,[23] yet the better the preparations for dealing effectively with it, the less likely terrorists are to think it worthwhile attempting in the first place.

An example of how preparation could help to deter was given by Richard Preston, author of *The Hot Zone* and *The Cobra Event*. Preston suggested that if smallpox were to be released anywhere in the US some 20-30 million people would have to be vaccinated quickly. There are only 7 million useable doses currently available, but he argued[24] that "[e]nough vaccine to protect the entire American population could be stored in a building smaller than a garage, and the vaccine would last for decades." Development of such a stockpile would, in his opinion, "pretty much remove smallpox from the arsenal of a terrorist."

A further example of the potential gains from sensible preparation is the development of simple oro-nasal masks which offer protection because the main route of attack with biological agents is through inhalation into the lungs. A recent study concluded[25] that "[m]asks that can reduce the potential effectiveness of BW agents by a factor of as much as 10,000 are available commercially, for less than $5 each." Although there are practical problems in getting excellent fit of such masks to the varied faces of large civilian populations, nevertheless, if they were available, and used, the consequences of a terrorist attack could be greatly diminished. International technical co-operation on mask development would again be to everyone's benefit.

An important factor favouring international response co-ordination in regard to terrorism is that it is quite likely that the consequences of an attack in one country could spread well beyond its borders. Another reason for co-operation is that there are widely differing levels of expertise and training in different countries.[26] International co-operation, particularly in the training of people who might have to deal with a terrorist attack, would be extremely beneficial.

Further international legal measures

Over the last four decades the number of international agreements directed at controlling terrorism has grown. These have come about in response to the perceived nature of possible terrorist attacks: for example, attacks on aircraft in the 1970s brought a series of agreements directed at various aspects of such terrorism.

The International Convention for the Suppression of Terrorist Bombings, which was opened for signature in January this year, specifically applies to biological and toxin agents. In the draft submitted by France on behalf of the Group of Seven (major industrialised countries) and Russia in February 1997,[27] a lethal device includes "any weapon or device that is intended, or has the capability, to cause death or serious bodily injury through the release, dissemination or impact of...biological agents or toxins". This surely reflects the developing international concern over terrorist use of such agents.

On a larger scale, as the *Christan Science Monitor* reported in mid-1997,[28] "[t]he builders are busy on the last great legal edifice of the 20th century: the International Criminal Court (ICC)." Recalling how the UN has expanded on the international law brought in with the post-Second World War Nuremberg trials, it was suggested that:

> *"The ICC will be the capstone of the legal structure....The ICC is to be permanent; its jurisdiction worldwide. Devised by treaty, it will be fully independent and funded by the treaty partners, who will also elect its 18 judges."*

Whilst the final outcome may be less than that envisaged in those high ideals, an agreement was signed in mid-July 1998 by 120 states.[29] The ICC will come into being in the not too distant future. What the court will do is provide a means by which the laws governing conduct in war — such as the Genocide Convention (Appendix 2) — can be put into practice by bringing those who violate them to justice. The medical profession has played an important role in developing the humanitarian law of war, particularly through the activities of the International Committee of the Red Cross. There is every reason to hope that their current efforts to develop the rules for prohibiting weapons which cause unnecessary suffering will eventually lead to better restrictions on the development of new weapons.[30]

Even when an International Criminal Court is brought into operation some authorities believe that it will still be necessary to have a Convention specifically to criminalise biological and chemical weapons.[31] The significant first article of the proposed 'Convention on the Prevention and Punishment of the Crime of Developing, Producing, Acquiring, Stockpiling, Retaining, Transferring or Using Biological or Chemical Weapons' is set out in Table 6.2. The accent on the responsibilities of individual people is noticeable, but so too, in 1(c), is the link with, and

Table 6.2: Draft Convention on the prevention and punishment of the crime of developing, producing, acquiring, stockpiling, retaining, transferring or using biological or chemical weapons*

Article I

1. Any person commits an offence if that person:

    a. orders, directs, plans or knowingly participates in the development, production, acquisition, stockpiling, retention, transfer or use of biological or chemical weapons; or

    b. attempts to commit any offence described in sub-paragraph (a); or

    c. assists, encourages or induces, in any way, anyone to engage in the development, production, acquisition, stockpiling, retention, transfer or use of biological or chemical weapons; or

    d. threatens to use biological or chemical weapons to cause death or injury to any person in order to compel a natural or legal person, international organization or State to do or refrain from doing any act.

2. It shall not be a defense against prosecution or extradition for the above offences that a person acted in an official capacity or under the orders or instruction of a State, a superior officer, a public or private authority or any other person or for any other reason.

3. Notwithstanding the above provisions of this Article, nothing in this Convention shall be construed as prohibiting activities that are not prohibited under the Chemical Weapons Convention or the Biological Weapons Convention or that are directed toward the fulfilment of a State's obligations under such conventions and that are conducted in accordance with its provisions.

*From [32]

constructive building upon, the Chemical Weapons Convention and the Biological and Toxin Weapons Convention.

There will clearly have to be a range of mechanisms by which the proliferation of biological weapons is constrained in the decades ahead. However, if a peaceful world governed by the rule of law is to come about, the balance will have to shift towards more integrated regulation, security and transparency obtained through an interlocking regime of international laws[33] and international institutions.[34]

The role of scientific specialists

At the end of his recent article on what might be done now, Richard Preston turned to a consideration of the role of scientific specialists:[35]

> "...The community of biologists in the United States has maintained hand-wringing silence on the ethics of creating bio-weapons — a reluctance to talk about it in public, even a disbelief that it is happening. Biological weapons are a disgrace to biology."

Wendy Barnaby came to similar conclusions here:[36]

> "I wrote to ten UK biological societies, asking them whether they had considered the developments in research that are relevant to biological warfare....Eight replied. None had considered BW in any depth..."

Preston argued that:[37]

> "Top biologists should assert their leadership and speak out, taking responsibility on behalf of their profession for the existence of these weapons and the means of protecting the population against them, just as leading physicists did a generation ago when nuclear weapons came along."

That would be a long-term project of considerable importance. A different comparison might be made with the recent landmines campaign, where a coalition of specialists, non-governmental organisations, some states and prominent individuals achieved a quite remarkable turnaround in public opinion and a new international agreement.[38] The latter comparison suggests a specific question of direct relevance now: what can the medical profession do to help strengthen the BTWC over the next one or two years?

The answer to that question will vary with the different opportunities available to individual members of the profession, but it is very important to recognise that present efforts to strengthen the Convention could easily fail, and that another opportunity might not arise until many more years of development of modern biotechnology have passed. Urgent action is required on at least two points. First, it is essential for the medical profession, and other scientific specialist groups like biologists, to be widely aware of this issue and that their professional organisations track the current negotiations and intervene if necessary. Second, it is vital that the medical profession reinforces the *central norm* — that these weapons are totally unacceptable — at every opportunity. That reinforcement may be the most significant contribution the profession can make in both the short and the longer term.

CHAPTER 7

Recommendations

The physician's role is the prevention and treatment of disease. The deliberate use of disease is directly contrary to the medical profession's whole ethos and rationale. Such misuse must be stigmatised so that it is completely rejected by civilised society.[1]

It has been stated that the future may well hold a 'Pandora's box of genetically engineered weapons'.[2] It is our duty to ensure that this particular Pandora's box remains closed to offensive state-sponsored programmes and terrorist organisations. The following recommendations for action and further research have been devised with this goal in mind.

The scientific and medical community

1. Professional scientists and physicians have an ethical responsibility to reinforce the central norm that biological and genetic weapons are unacceptable. This should be explicitly stated in codes of professional conduct in order to safeguard the public interest in matters of health and safety.

2. The potential for malign use of biotechnology places an ethical responsibility on the medical and scientific community to protect the integrity of their work. Developments should be closely monitored, and openly debated, particularly in

relation to the potential use of genome mapping for eugenicist or genocidal purposes.

3. The World Health Organization's disease reporting network should be expanded, particularly in relation to unexplained outbreaks of disease which could potentially arise from the development or use of biological or genetic weapons. Pressure should be exerted to ensure full participation of medical staff in all nation states.

4. Medical education courses should be available to familiarise medical professionals with the signs of biological warfare-related disease — this may encourage a mindset which enables future healthcare professionals to observe and identify the unexpected.

5. The recent success of the anti-landmines campaign has signalled the importance of public education campaigns regarding the development of ethical arms policies. Reports such as this one should be actively promoted to stimulate public debate on the ethical and scientific issues surrounding biotechnology and its possible uses in warfare.

International action

6. The international community should aim to strengthen the prohibitive norms of the 1925 Geneva Protocol and the 1972 Biological and Toxin Weapons Convention (BTWC).

7. The Biological and Toxin Weapons Convention should be strengthened to improve verification procedures and provide measures to promote compliance with the agreement. We believe that the measures being considered in the Ad Hoc Group are likely to be the most effective means of establishing such controls. These measures place an ethical responsibility

on anyone who may have information on the trafficking or development of biological agents.

8. The international bioscientific community should support colleagues formerly employed on biological weapons programmes (eg the countries of the Former Soviet Union), but who are now unemployed or underemployed. The UN should work with nations/national governments including the G8 group of countries on methods to help weapons laboratories convert to peaceful purposes. Such measures should aim to decrease the numbers of disaffected scientists who may otherwise be tempted to perform illicit biological weapons-related research for proliferant nations or terrorist groups.

9. Internet service providers have an ethical obligation to ensure that information on how to make biological weapons is not available on their websites. Consideration should be given to how this duty could be legislatively reinforced.

10. The developed world should promote national security and equality in social relations in underdeveloped nations through effective aid policies and ethical investment, to prevent extremes of hostility, fanaticism and alienation escalating into biological terrorism or warfare.

National government agencies

11. In the interests of national security, Governments should closely monitor activities within their own and other countries under which doctors may be pressured into working on biological weapons programmes and take appropriate actions where there is evidence that this is taking place.

12. Governments should consider a 'web of deterrence' to prevent biological warfare being used as a terrorist weapon. This

should include epidemiological and medical training and expanded clinical facilities to respond to the potential threats. The early detection of a potential hazard will be aided by the expansion of online databases reporting unexplained outbreaks of disease.

13. The 'web of deterrence' should include initiatives from national governments to build a consensus in civil society against the use of biological weapons, which should involve religious and cultural leaders.

14. There is no feasible medical response to innovative and unknown biological weapons — prevention of their development and production is the only valid civil defence measure. However, it is recognised that there should be civil defence preparation for small-scale attacks with known biological agents.

15. Disease control and surveillance measures should be enhanced to aid early detection of pathogens, and extra resources should be made available for research into early warning and identification of biological warfare agents.

16. Every country should have an appropriate national inspectorate to carry out regular inspections of the premises of pharmaceutical manufacturers, and those who routinely handle biohazardous material, to monitor the nature of biological and genetic research.

17. A warning list of dual-use material and equipment (ie material and equipment that could be used by other nations/terrorist organisations to develop biological weapons) should be made available to industry and regulatory bodies to assist ethical export decisions, on a worldwide basis.

Biological weapons

In the course of evolution a range of pathogens has come to attack human beings, their animals and plant crops. In the past, large, offensive, biological weapons programmes considered attacks on animals and plants and though the potential effectiveness of animal and plant pathogens is clear, for example from the lengths to which we go to keep foot and mouth disease out of the UK and from the history of the Irish potato famine in the last century, most biological warfare programmes involved consideration of attacks on people. The production, and potential use, of biological weapons remains a great danger.

Micro-organisms — bacteria, fungi and viruses — attack people by a variety of mechanisms. These sometimes involve the production of damaging, non-living, chemical toxins. Toxins are therefore covered by both the Chemical Weapons Convention and the Biological and Toxin Weapons Convention (BTWC). An attacker can also disrupt bodily functions by producing imbalances in naturally occurring substances such as peptides, so misuse of such other agents is also covered by the BTWC. Naturally-occurring pathogens provide a variety of options for a military planner. There are lethal agents (pathogens) such as anthrax or basically incapacitating agents such as Q-fever; there are agents which are highly contagious such as plague or agents such as anthrax which are unlikely to cause an epidemic after first use. In nature, pathogens have evolved to attack human beings in a variety of different ways, such as through contaminated water or insect vectors. Clearly, some such routes could be considered in, for example, a sabotage campaign.

Since the early French studies of the 1920s, and particularly since the British studies during the second World War, it has been clear that some agents have characteristics such as stability in the environment which allow for the kind of large-scale use necessary for military effectiveness. The preferred mode of infection is through inhalation of the agent into the lungs. Studies on anthrax showed that it was possible to produce a cloud of the agent with particles of the correct size and concentration to be inhaled in sufficient quantities to produce reliable infection of people over a very wide area. With the difficulty of detecting use of the agent, and the probability of rapid death without treatment, anthrax has been an obvious choice in offensive biological weapons programmes. Given its toxicity, botulinum toxin has been another obvious choice. The challenge for the military planner is therefore to find a means of producing, stockpiling and delivering the agent to the target in the face of the living organism's fragility. This problem has been solved in research and development programmes where dried agent in cluster bombs, line-source generators and even multiple missile warheads have been shown to be effective means of reliable delivery. A particularly important development has been the growing understanding of the behaviour of micro-organisms in air — aerobiology. In addition, the increasing understanding of weather patterns has helped to give confidence in the predictability of attack effects.

Appendix 2

International arms control

Independent political entities have often found it expedient to agree means of regulating armaments — for example, in peace treaties following wars. As the application of science and technology to the industrialisation of warfare has led to ever more destructive weaponry spreading around the globe, the need to regulate armaments has become more and more pressing. A significant part of the enormous growth in international law over the last century has been concerned with arms control and disarmament. The Nuclear Non-Proliferation Treaty (NPT) and the Conventional Forces in Europe (CFE) Treaty are major examples of such stabilisation processes.

It cannot be argued, however, that arms control and disarmament agreements arise simply from the need to regulate armaments. International arms control agreements partly result from other political considerations in inter-state negotiations and also from *intra*-state (and often intra-alliance) concerns. With this level of complexity, a window of opportunity rarely occurs where a particular agreement can be reached. Additionally, for an agreement on significant weapons system to be achieved, it has to be accepted by the military establishments of major powers. Once an agreement is reached, however, states are expected to, and usually do, live up to their undertakings. To do otherwise would be to risk losing credibility in other international dealings.

Arms control agreements can be made bilaterally, as they frequently were by the two superpowers during the Cold War, or multilaterally between a number of different nations. Multilateral negotiations frequently take place within the United Nations system where the Conference on Disarmament in Geneva provides the forum for discussions. When an agreement is reached in negotiations, the states that wish to become parties sign the agreement, and then proceed through their national (internal) ratification processes. The agreement enters into force when conditions agreed in the negotiations — such as a specified minimum number of individual state ratifications — are satisfied.

International arms control agreements have a number of standard clauses, for example allowing for review or amendment of the agreement. It is also possible to agree to leave the original agreement intact, but to add a protocol to it. This is what is presently happening in regard to the Biological and Toxin Weapons Convention (BTWC). The BTWC Protocol will be subject to ratification by the States Parties in the same way as the original treaty, and there will be agreed provisions for its entry into force. Although it is to be expected that states will abide by their undertakings as a matter of self-interest, it is not surprising, when national security is involved, that proper verification is also required to ensure that parties are living up to their obligations. In order to *achieve* verification of complex multilateral agreements, it is vital that some organisation is set up to oversee the operation of any agreement when it enters into force. Complex arms control agreements will continue to be developed to regulate new forms of weaponry well into the future. The presently still-cumbersome methods of negotiation may be systematised and streamlined as the evolution of law-making progresses.

The international humanitarian law of war is concerned with the conduct of warfare: how the victims of war such as the wounded and prisoners are treated, and the kinds of weapons that may be used. It has proved easier to develop the law concerned with the treatment of victims through the Geneva Conventions than to develop restrictions on weapons. However, in recent years we have seen determined efforts to improve the restrictions on weapons, such as on anti-personnel landmines. There is an intimate connection between the international humanitarian law of war and the international agreement of measures for arms control and disarmament. Warfare is the result of a breakdown in the normal peaceful and legal means of state behaviour. In such circumstances it is always possible that there will be resort to measures considered unacceptable in peacetime, but weapons that have not previously been integrated into military forces are less likely to be used if warfare does break out.

Appendix 3

Pathogens and toxins

Extracts from Annex A.II lists and criteria (agents and toxins) of BWC/Ad Hoc Group/38*

Human pathogens

The following list of human pathogens and toxins was discussed by the Group and recognized to be relevant for developing a list or lists of bacteriological (biological) agents and toxins for specific measures to strengthen the Convention:

I. Natural organisms

Viruses

1   Crimean-Congo haemorrhagic fever virus

2   Eastern equine encephalitis virus

3   Ebola virus

4   Hantaviruses

5   Japanese encephalitis virus

6   Junin virus

7   Lassa fever virus

8   Machupo virus

9   Marburg virus

10   Rift Valley Virus

11   Tick-borne encephalitis virus

12   Variola virus (Smallpox virus)

13   Venezuelan equine encephalitis virus

14   Western equine encephalitis virus

15   Yellow fever virus

16   Kyasanur Forest Disease virus

Bacteria

1   *Bacillus anthracis*

2   *Brucella spp*

3   *Chlamydia psittaci*

4   *Clostridium botulinum*

5   *Francisella tularensis (tularemia)*

6   *Pseudomonas (Burkholderia) mallei*

7   *Pseudomonas (Burkholderia) pseudomallei*

8   *Yersinia pestis*

Rickettsiae

1   *Coxiella burnetti*

2   *Rickettsia prowazekii*

3   *Rickettsia rickettsii*

Fungi

1   *Histoplasma capsulatum* (incl. var *duboisii*)

II. New organisms resulting from genetic manipulations

III. Molecular agents

Toxins

1   Abrin (*A. precatorius*)

2   Botulinum toxins (*Clostridium botulinum*)

3   *Clostridium perfringens* (tox)

4   *Corynebacterium diphteriae* (tox)

5   Cyanginosins (Microcystins) (*Microcystis aeruginosa*)

6   Enterotoxins (*Staphylococcus aureus*)

7   Ricin (*Ricinus communis*)

8   Saxitoxin (*Ganyaulax catanella*)

9   Shigatoxin (*Shigella dysenteriae*)

10   Tetanus toxin (*Clostridium tetani*)

11   Tetrodotoxin (*Spheroides rufripes*)

12   Trichothecene mycotoxins

13   Verrucologen (*Myrothecium verrucaria*)

14   Aflatoxins

IV. Other agents

Animal pathogens

The following list of animal pathogens was discussed by the Group for further consideration with a view to developing a future list or lists of bacteriological (biological) agents and toxins, where relevant, for specific measures designed to strengthen the Convention:

I. Natural organisms

1   African swine fever virus

2   Avian influenza virus (Fowl plague virus)

3   Bluetongue virus

4   Camel pox virus

5   Classic swine fever virus (Hog cholera virus)

6   Contagious bovine (pleuropneumonia)/*Mycoplasma mycoides var. mycoides*

7   Contagious caprine (pleuropneumonia)/*Mycoplasma mycoides var. capri*

8   Foot and mouth virus

9   Herpes B virus (monkey)

10 Newcastle disease virus

11 Peste des petits ruminants virus

12 Porcine enterovirus type 9

13 Rabies virus

14 Rinderpest virus (Cattle plague virus)

15 Sheep pox virus

16 Teschen disease virus

17 Vesicular stomatitis virus

18 African horse sickness virus

19 Swine vesicular disease virus

II. New organisms resulting from genetic manipulation

III. Molecular agents

IV. Other agents

Plant pathogens

The following list of plant pathogens was discussed by the Group for further consideration with a view to developing a future list or lists of bacteriological (biological) agents and toxins, where relevant, for specific measures designed to strengthen the Convention:

I. Natural organisms

1   Citrus greening disease bacteria

2   *Colletotrichum coffeanum var. Virulans*

3   *Chochliobolus miyabeanus*

4   *Dothistroma pini (Scirrhia pini)*

5   *Erwinia amylovora*

6   *Microcyclus ulei*

7   *Phytophthora infestans*

8   *Pseudomonas solanacearum*

9   *Puccinia erianthi*

10 *Puccinia graminis*

11 *Puccinia striiformiis (Puccinia glumarum)*

12 *Pyricularia oryzae*

13 Sugar cane Fiji disease virus

14 *Tilletia indica*

15 *Ustilago maydis*

16 *Xanthomonas albilineans*

17 *Xanthomonas campestris pv citri*

18 *Xanthomonas campestris pv oryzae*

19 *Sclerotinia sclerotiorum*

20 *Thrips palmi Karny*

21 *Frankliniella occidentalis*

II. New organisms resulting from genetic manipulation

III. Molecular agents

IV. Other agents

114

Definition of selected terms

Natural organisms: Bacteria, viruses, funguses, rickettsiae, chlamydias, mycoplasmas, protozoa, insects and any other living organisms which, owing to their characteristics and in accordance with the selection criteria, could be used as biological weapons.

New organisms resulting from genetic manipulation: Organisms whose genetic material has been altered using genetic manipulation techniques. The following must be included:

(a) Genetically modified organisms containing nucleic acid sequences associated with the pathogenicity derived from listed agents;

(b) Genetically modified organisms containing nucleic acid sequences coding for any of the listed molecular agents;

(c) Genetically modified organisms containing nucleic acid sequences associated with the pathogenicity of agents classified in risk groups 3 and 4 (in accordance with the criteria set out in the 1993 WHO Laboratory Biosafety Handbook), which are not necessarily listed;

(d) Genetically modified organisms which, owing to their new characteristics, would fall in risk groups 3 and 4 (in accordance with the criteria set out in the 1993 WHO Laboratory Biosafety Handbook).

Molecular agents: Toxins, bioregulators or chemical substances of biological origin.

Other agents: Prions (at the stage of research, development and production, excluding diagnostic activities) and any other new agent not included in the previous groups.

*Source: United Nations. (1997). Procedural Report of the Ad Hoc Group of the States Parties to the Convention on the Prohibition of the Development, Production and Stockpiling of Bacteriological (Biological) and Toxin Weapons and on Their Destruction. Eighth Session, BWC/AD HOC GROUP/38, 6 October. Geneva: United Nations.

Glossary

Aerobiology: the study of airborne micro-organisms, pollen spores, seeds or infectious agents.

Alleles: alternative versions of the same gene, or DNA sequence occupying equivalent positions on homologous (pairs of) chromosomes.

Anthrax: infectious disease affecting humans and animals caused by *Bacillus anthracis*. The disease can take three main forms in humans — cutaneous, pulmonary and intestinal.

Antisense oligonucleotides: short stretches of nucleotides which contain the opposite coding sequence to a specific mRNA transcript used in the cell to make a protein. Oligonucleotides can bind to the complimentary mRNA transcript, preventing the production of its protein product.

Benign microorganisms: minute living organisms which do not cause virulent or fatal disease.

Biological and Toxin Weapons Convention 1975 (BTWC): signed at Washington, London and Moscow on 10 April 1972, and entered into force 26 March 1975 and now has 140 member countries. The convention prohibits the development, production and stockpiling of bacteriological (biological) and toxin weapons. At present lacks any effective verification provisions to ensure that states are living up to their undertakings.

Biological warfare: use of disease-producing agents, such as bacteria and viruses, as weapons targeted at humans, animals or plants.

Biological diversity: the variety of life forms in a particular habitat.

Bioregulatory peptides: peptides involved in regulating metabolic pathways.

Biotechnology: the industrial application of techniques and instruments of research (particularly those associated with genetic engineering) in the biological sciences.

Bioterrorist: a terrorist using disease producing agents such as bacteria and viruses as a weapon.

Chemical Weapons Convention (CWC): a modern (1993) arms control agreement which effectively bans chemical weapons and includes strict verification provisions. Entered into force on 29 April 1997 with 165 signatories.

Chromosome: a structure primarily composed of the DNA that carries the genetic information of the cell.

Deletion mutations: the loss or absence of a section of DNA or part of a chromosome.

DNA: deoxyribonucleic acid, molecular structure found in living cells which codes genetic information for the transmission of inherited traits.

DNA bases: four chemicals called adenine, guanine, cytosine and thymine which form part of the DNA molecule. They are linked together by sugar (deoxyribose) and phosphate groups to form a strand of DNA. The order in which the bases are linked forms the DNA code which carried the genetic information.

DNA fingerprinting: a method for revealing unique patterns in certain regions of an individual's DNA which has forensic and other uses in identification. Certain sequences are repeated in the DNA. The repeated sequences are unique to any one individual (with the exception of identical twins).

Dual-use technology: technology which has both civil and military uses.

Enzyme: a biological catalyst which hastens or brings about a chemical reaction within a cell without itself being consumed in the process of the reaction.

Ethnic group: a social group or category of the population that, in larger society, is set apart and bound together by common ties of race, language, nationality or culture. They may also have shared genetic characteristics which make them more vulnerable — or exclusively susceptible — to particular diseases or biological attack.

Eugenics: an attempt to eliminate undesirable qualities from the human race by selective breeding and genetic modification.

Forensic science: the application of science to legal questions.

Gene: unit of hereditary information that occupies a fixed position in a chromosome and directs the synthesis of proteins.

Genetic map: a map of the location of the genes for various inherited characteristics in the chromosomes.

Genetic/ethnic weapons: weapons which may be used to target biological agents on particular genetic or ethnic groups.

Genetic modification: the production of new combinations of genetic material by altering the DNA of an organism.

Genotype: the total genetic information contained in a cell.

Glanders: infectious and contagious disease affecting horses, which may infect humans and most frequently occurs through occupational contact with diseased horses.

Homo Sapiens: genus and species to which all modern human beings belong.

Human Genome Project: international scientific project to sequence the 3,000 million DNA bases in human DNA, which provide the biological instructions to make a human being.

Immune system: the biological defence system, which protects the body from disease-causing microorganisms and other foreign (non-self) substances.

Microbial pathogenesis: disease process caused by microorganisms.

Microencapsulation: in biological warfare — the coating of fragile agents to allow them to be more effectively delivered by conventional means.

Minisatellites: Short sequences of DNA which are each repeated 10-100 times, one after the other. The number of repeat units in each minisatellite is very variable. Relatives may share the same number of repeat units in some minisatellites, but not others.

mRNA: messenger RNA (ribonucleic acid). A copy of a gene, made from RNA, which is transported out of the nucleus where it is used to direct the synthesis of a specific protein.

Neuroscience: study of functional or organic disorders of the nervous system.

Nucleic acid: collective term for DNA or RNA. Each type of nucleic acid is composed of a string of nucleotides which consist of three elements, a base, a sugar and a phosphate group.

Nucleotide: any member of a class of organic compounds in which the molecular structure comprises a nitrogen-containing unit (base) linked to a sugar and phosphate group.

pH tolerance: measured ability to withstand acidity of aqueous or other liquid solutions.

Polymorphism: structural or functional variations among members of a single species.

Proliferant nations: a general term used to categorise states thought to be near to obtaining, or just having obtained, a dangerous weapon of mass destruction.

Prophylactic: any act, drug, procedure, or equipment which guards against a negative outcome (eg death or disease).

Recombinant DNA techniques: ways of regrouping genes or transplanting genes from one chromosome to another using advances in biotechnology.

Ribozyme: an RNA molecule capable of acting as an enzyme.

SIrUS project: an initiative involving an expert panel convened by the International Committee of the Red Cross to determine which weapons cause 'superfluous injury or unnecessary suffering', to facilitate their prohibition. The findings were published in 1998 and medical organisations and associations have been invited to endorse its findings.

Sporulation: the production or release of spores.

Tropism: an automatic movement made by an organism towards or away from a source of stimulation.

United Nations Special Commission (UNSCOM): The UN Special Commission on Iraq. A subsidiary organ of the Security Council entrusted with the task of implementing the disarming of Iraq according to the ceasefire resolution following the 1991 Gulf War and with the continuing monitoring of Iraq's weapons capability.

Verification Protocol (to the BTWC): an addition to the Biological and Toxin Weapons Convention currently being negotiated with the aim of adding effective verification measures to ensure the State Parties live up to their undertakings.

Viral vectors: viruses which can act as a vehicle for DNA, eg genetically modified DNA. They allow the DNA to be transferred to other organisms.

Virology: a branch of microbiology dealing with the study of viruses.

References

Chapter 1

1   British Medical Association. (1983). *The Medical Effects of Nuclear War*. Chichester: Wiley.

2   British Medical Association. (1988). *Nuclear Attack: Ethics and Casualty Section*. London: BMA.

3   British Medical Association. (1987). *The Medical Implications of Chemical and Biological Warfare*. London: BMA.

4   Coupland R (Ed.). (1997). *The SIrUS Project: towards a determination of which weapons cause "superfluous injury or unnecessary suffering"*. Geneva: International Committee of the Red Cross.

5   Redmond C. *et al.* (1998). Deadly relic of the Great War. *Nature*, 393, 747-8.

6   Dando MR. (1994). *Biological Warfare in the 21st Century: Biotechnology and the Proliferation of Biological Weapons*. London: Brassey's.

7   Zilinskas RA. (1997). Iraq's biological weapons: The past as future. *Journal of the American Medical Association*, 275, 418-24.

8   Preston R. (1998). Annals of warfare: The bioweaponeers. *New Yorker*, March, pp. 52-65.

9   International Committee of the Red Cross. (1996). *The Medical Profession and the Effects of Weapons: Report of the Symposium, Montreux, March, 1996*. Geneva: ICRC.

10 World Medical Association. (1996). *Statement: Weapons and their Relation to Life and Health*. 48th WMA General Assembly, 20-26 October, Somerset West, South Africa.

11 Fidler DP. (1998). *War and Infectious Diseases: International Law and the Public Health Consequences of Armed Conflict*. Paper presented at the First International Conference on Addressing Environmental Consequences of War: Legal, Economic and Scientific Perspectives, June 10-12, Smithsonian Institute, Washington, DC.

12 United Nations. (1985). *The United Nations and Disarmament: 1945-1985*. New York: United Nations.

Chapter 2

1   Poupard JA. and Miller LA. (1992). History of biological warfare: Catapults to capsomeres. *Annals of the New York Academy of Sciences, 666,* 9-19.

2   Wheelis M. (1998) Biological warfare before 1914: The prescientific era. In E Geissler and JE van Courtland Moon (Eds.), *Biological and Toxin Weapons Research, Development and Use from the Middle Ages to 1945: A Critical Comparative Analysis.* Oxford: Oxford University Press, (for SIPRI). In press.

3   Wheelis M. (1998). Biological warfare before 1914: The prescientific era. In E Geissler and JE van Courtland Moon (Eds.), *Biological and Toxin Weapons Research, Development and Use from the Middle Ages to 1945: A Critical Comparative Analysis.* Oxford: Oxford University Press, (for SIPRI). In press.

4   van Courtland Moon, J. (1993). Controlling chemical and biological weapons through World War II. In RD Burns (Ed.), *Encyclopedia of Arms Control and Disarmament,* Volume II. New York: Charles Scribner's Sons.

5   Dando MR. (1998). The development of international legal constraints on biological warfare in the 20th century. *Finnish Yearbook of International Law 1998.* In press.

6   Boserup A. (1973). *The Problem of Chemical and Biological Warfare: Volume III CBW and the Law of War.* Stockholm: Almqvist and Wiksell, (for SIPRI).

7   Poupard JA, Miller LA. (1992). History of biological warfare: Catapults to capsomeres. *Annals of the New York Academy of Sciences, 666,* 9-19.

8   Wheelis M. (1998) Biological warfare before 1914: The prescientific era. In E Geissler and JE van Courtland Moon (Eds.), *Biological and Toxin Weapons Research, Development and Use from the Middle Ages to 1945: A Critical Comparative Analysis.* Oxford: Oxford University Press, (for SIPRI). In press.

9   Wheelis M. (1998) Biological sabotage in the First World War. In E Geissler and JE van Courtland Moon (Eds.), *Biological and Toxin Weapons Research, Development and Use from the Middle Ages to 1945: A Critical Comparative Analysis.* Oxford: Oxford University Press, (for SIPRI). In press.

10 Wheelis M. (1998) Biological sabotage in the First World War. In E Geissler and JE van Courtland Moon (Eds.), *Biological and Toxin Weapons Research, Development and Use from the Middle Ages to 1945: A Critical Comparative Analysis.* Oxford: Oxford University Press, (for SIPRI). In press.

11 Lepick O. (1998). French activities related to biological warfare: 1919-1945. In E Geissler and JE van Courtland Moon (Eds.), *Biological and Toxin Weapons Research, Development and Use from the Middle Ages to 1945: A Critical Comparative Analysis.* Oxford: Oxford University Press, (for SIPRI). In press.

12 Wheelis M. (1998) Biological sabotage in the First World War. In E Geissler and JE van Courtland Moon (Eds.), *Biological and Toxin Weapons Research, Development and Use from the Middle Ages to 1945: A Critical Comparative Analysis.* Oxford: Oxford University Press, (for SIPRI). In press.

13   Dando MR. (1998). The development of international legal constraints on biological warfare in the 20th century. *Finnish Yearbook of International Law 1998*. In press.

14   Dando MR. (1998). The development of international legal constraints on biological warfare in the 20th century. *Finnish Yearbook of International Law 1998*. In press.

15   Goldblat J. (1996) *Arms Control: A Guide to Negotiations and Agreements*. London: Sage, (for PRIO).

16   Faludi Col. G. (1997). *Challenges of BW Control and Defence During Arms Reduction*. Paper presented to a NATO Advanced Research Workshop on 'Conversion of Former BW Facilities', November, Budapest.

17   Mobley James A, Col USAR. (1995). Biological Warfare in the Twentieth Century: Lessons from the past, challenges for the future. Military Medicine, 160, 547-53.

18   Harris SH. (1994). *Factories of Death: Japanese Biological Warfare 1932-45 and the American Cover Up*. London: Routledge.

19   Harris SH. (1992). Japanese biological warfare research on humans: A case study of microbiology and ethics. *Annals of the New York Academy of Sciences, 666, 21-45*.

20   Gold H. (1996). *Unit 731 Testimony: Japan's Wartime Human Experimentation Program*. Tokyo: Yenbooks.

21   Scientific and Technical Advisory Section GHQ, AFPAC. (1945). *Report on Scientific Intelligence Survey in Japan (September & October 1945). Volume V — Biological Warfare*. Report No. BIOS/JAP/PR/746. British Intelligence Objectives Sub-Committee. London: HMSO.

22   Ismay HL. (1942). 'Japanese Attempts at Bacteriological Warfare in China'. Note from Office of Minister of Defence to Prime Minister, 9th July. In Public Record Office File PREMIER 3/65/5119. London: Public Record Office.

23   Harris SH. (1994). *Factories of Death: Japanese Biological Warfare 1932-45 and the American Cover Up*. London: Routledge.

24   Harris SH. (1992). Japanese biological warfare research on humans: A case study of microbiology and ethics. *Annals of the New York Academy of Sciences, 666, 21-45*.

25   Gold H. (1996). *Unit 731 Testimony: Japan's Wartime Human Experimentation Program*. Tokyo: Yenbooks.

26   Harris SH. (1992). Japanese biological warfare research on humans: A case study of microbiology and ethics. *Annals of the New York Academy of Sciences, 666, 21-45*.

27   Scientific and Technical Advisory Section GHQ, AFPAC. (1945). *Report on Scientific Intelligence Survey in Japan (September & October 1945). Volume V — Biological Warfare*. Report No. BIOS/JAP/PR/746. British Intelligence Objectives Sub-Committee. London: HMSO.

28   Barnes Major JM et al. (1945). *A Review of German Activities in the Field of Biological Warfare*. Intelligence Report No. B-C-H-H/305. Washington DC: War Department, ALSOS Mission, 12 September.

29   Carter GB. (1992). *Porton Down: 75 Years of Chemical and Biological Research*. London: HMSO.

30   Carter GB. (1992). Biological warfare and biological defence in the United Kingdom 1940- 1979. *Journal of the Royal United Services Institute*, December, 67-74.

31   DERA. 'The history of DERA — Porton Down'. www.dra.hmg.gb/html/who_are/history/porturi.htm.

32   Carter GB. (1992). Biological warfare and biological defence in the United Kingdom 1940- 1979. *Journal of the Royal United Services Institute*, December, 67-74.

33   Carter GB. (1992). Biological warfare and biological defence in the United Kingdom 1940- 1979. *Journal of the Royal United Services Institute*, December, 67-74.

34   Dando MR. (1994). *Biological Warfare in the 21st Century: Biotechnology and the Proliferation of Biological Weapons*. London: Brassey's.

35   Carter GB. and Pearson GS. (1996). North Atlantic chemical and biological research collaboration: 1916-1995. *Journal of Strategic Studies*, 19, 74-103.

36   Millward D. (1996). Allies drew up plans to poison German crops. *The Daily Telegraph*, 8 January, pp. 2.

37   Joint Technical Warfare Committee. (1945). *Potentialities of Weapons of War During the Next Ten Years*. TWC (45) 42, 12 November.

38   Carter GB. (1992). Biological warfare and biological defence in the United Kingdom 1940- 1979. *Journal of the Royal United Services Institute*, December, 67-74.

39   Joint Technical Warfare Committee. (1945). *Potentialities of Weapons of War During the Next Ten Years*. TWC (45) 42, 12 November.

40   Dando MR. (1994). *Biological Warfare in the 21st Century: Biotechnology and the Proliferation of Biological Weapons*. London: Brassey's.

41   Miller DL. (1952). *History of Air Force Participation in Biological Warfare Program 1944- 1951*. Historical Study No. 194. Historical Office, Office of the Executive, Air Materiel Command, Wright-Patterson Air Force Base, September.

42   Creasy Col WM. (1950). *Biological Warfare*. Presentation to the Secretary of Defense's Ad Hoc Committee on CEBAR, 24 February.

43   US Army. (1973). *Joint CB Technical Data Source Book: Volume VIII Bacterial Diseases: Part Two Anthrax*. DTC 73-27. Headquarters Test and Evaluation Command, Deseret Test Center, Fort Douglas, Utah.

44   Bernstein B. (1990). Origins of the US biological warfare program. In S Wright (Ed.), *Preventing a Biological Arms Race*. Cambridge, Mass: MIT Press.

45   US Army. (1977). *US Army Activity in the US Biological Warfare Programs*. Volumes I and II. Department of the Army, Washington DC, 24 February.

46   US Army. (1977). *US Army Activity in the US Biological Warfare Programs*. Volumes I and II. Department of the Army, Washington DC, 24 February.

47   US Army. (1977). *US Army Activity in the US Biological Warfare Programs*. Volumes I and II. Department of the Army, Washington DC, 24 February.

48   United States. (1949). *Report of the Secretary of Defense's Ad Hoc Committee on Biological Warfare*. JCS, 2C934, 11 July.

49 Perry Robinson J. (1991). *Adherence to the 1972 Biological Weapons Convention*. Paper presented at the Quaker Residential Conference on 'Strengthening the Biological Weapons Convention', 31 May-2 June, Chateau de Bessey, Switzerland.

50 Dando MR. (1994). *Biological Warfare in the 21st Century: Biotechnology and the Proliferation of Biological Weapons*. London: Brassey's.

51 US Army. (1977). *US Army Activity in the US Biological Warfare Programs*. Volumes I and II. Department of the Army, Washington DC, 24 February.

52 Miller DL. (1952). *History of Air Force Participation in Biological Warfare Program 1944-1951*. Historical Study No. 194. Historical Office, Office of the Executive, Air Materiel Command, Wright-Patterson Air Force Base, September.

53 Dando MR. (1994). *Biological Warfare in the 21st Century: Biotechnology and the Proliferation of Biological Weapons*. London: Brassey's.

54 Carter GB. (1992). Biological warfare and biological defence in the United Kingdom 1940-1979. *Journal of the Royal United Services Institute*, December, 67-74.

55 Dasey CF. (1990). Medical benefits of the Biological Defense Research Program. *Politics and the Life Sciences*, 9, 77-84.

56 King J and Strauss H. (1990). The hazards of defensive biological warfare programs. In S Wright (Ed.), *Preventing a Biological Arms Race*. Cambridge, Mass: MIT Press.

57 United Nations. (1969). *Chemical and Bacteriological (Biological) Weapons and the Effects of Their Possible Use*. E.69.1.24. New York: United Nations.

58 World Health Organization. (1970). *Health Aspects of Chemical and Biological Weapons*. Geneva: WHO.

59 Dando MR. (1994). *Biological Warfare in the 21st Century: Biotechnology and the Proliferation of Biological Weapons*. London: Brassey's.

60 US Army Medical Research Institute of Infectious Diseases. (1994). *Biological Weapons Proliferation: Technical Report*. DNA-MIPR-90-715. Washington DC: Department of the Army.

61 Office of Technology Assessment. (1993). *Proliferation of Weapons of Mass Destruction: Assessing the Risks*. OTA-ISC-559, August. United States Congress.

62 Office of Technology Assessment. (1993). *Proliferation of Weapons of Mass Destruction: Assessing the Risks*. OTA-ISC-559, August. United States Congress.

63 Central Intelligence Agency. (1996). Responses for the Record (10 May). Hearings on *Current and Projected National Security Threats to the United States and its Interests Abroad*. Select Committee on Intelligence, United States Senate, One Hundred and Fourth Congress, Second Session, 22 February.

64 Secretary General. (1995). *Report of the Secretary General on the Status of the Implementation of the Special Commission's Plan for the Ongoing Monitoring and Verification of Iraq's Compliance with the Relevant Parts of Section C of Security Council Resolution 687 (1991)*. S/1995/864. New York: United Nations.

65 Zilinskas RA. (1997). Iraq's biological weapons: The past as future. *Journal of the American Medical Association*, 278, 418-24.

66   Adams JR. (1998) Iraq's yellow rain: The weapons behind the latest crisis. *The American Spectator*, March, pp. 1-5. (from the WorldWideWeb at http://www. amspec.org:80/archives/98-03_adams.html.).

67   Abramova FA. *et al.* (1993). Pathology of inhalation anthrax in 42 cases from the Sverdlovsk outbreak of 1979. *Proc. Natl. Acad. Sci. USA*, 90, 2291-4.

68   Jackson PJ *et al.* (1998). PCR analysis of tissue samples from the 1979 Sverdlovsk anthrax victims: The presence of multiple *Bacillus anthracis* strains in different victims. *Proc. Natl. Acad. Sci. USA*, 95, 1224-9.

69   Leitenberg M. (1996). *Biological Weapons Arms Control*. Project on Rethinking Arms Control, Center for International and Security Studies at Maryland. PRAC Paper No. 16, May. University of Maryland at College Park, Maryland, USA.

70   Steinbrunner JD. (1998). Biological weapons: A plague upon all houses. *Foreign Policy*, Winter 1997-98, 85-96.

71   Sawyer D. (1998). *Germ Warfare: Weapons of Terror*. Script of *Prime Time*, ABC News, 1-38, 25 February.

72   Nicolson GL and Nicolson NL. (1997). The eight myths of Operation 'Desert Storm' and Gulf War Syndrome. *Medicine, Conflict and Survival*, 13, 140-6.

73   Poupard JA, Miller LA. (1992). History of biological warfare: Catapults to capsomeres. *Annals of the New York Academy of Sciences*, 666, 9-19.

74   Sopko JF. (1997). The changing proliferation threat. *Foreign Policy*, Winter 1996-97, 3-19.

75   Leklem E and Boulden L. (1997). Exorcising Project B: Pretoria probes its shady chemical past. *Jane's Intelligence Review*, August, 372-5.

76   Carus WS. (1997). *The Threat of Bioterrorism*. Strategic Forum No. 127. Institute of National Strategic Studies, National Defense University, Washington DC.

77   Carus WS. (1997). *The Threat of Bioterrorism*. Strategic Forum No. 127. Washington DC: Institute of National Strategic Studies, National Defense University.

78   Betts RK. (1998). The new threat of mass destruction. *Foreign Affairs*, 77, 26-41.

79   Franz Col DR *et al.* (1997). Clinical recognition and management of patients exposed to biological warfare agents. *Journal of the American Medical Association*, 278, 399-411.

80   Wheelis M. (1997). *Addressing the Full Range of Biological Warfare in a BWC Compliance Protocol*. Paper presented at Pugwash Meeting No. 229, 'Strengthening the Biological Weapons Convention', 20-21 September, Geneva.

81   Wheelis M. (1997). *Addressing the Full Range of Biological Warfare in a BWC Compliance Protocol*. Paper presented at Pugwash Meeting No. 229, 'Strengthening the Biological Weapons Convention', 20-21 September, Geneva.

82   Wheelis M. (1997). *Addressing the Full Range of Biological Warfare in a BWC Compliance Protocol*. Paper presented at Pugwash Meeting No. 229, 'Strengthening the Biological Weapons Convention', 20-21 September, Geneva.

83   Leitenberg M. (1997). The desirability of international sanctions against false allegations of use of biological weapons. *The Monitor: Nonproliferation, Demilitarization and Arms Control*, Fall 1997/Winter 1998, 39-46.

84   Dando MR. (1996). *A New Form of Warfare: The Rise of Non-Lethal Weapons.* London: Brassey's.

85   Ministry of Defence press release. 'Microbiologist appointed to review south coast defence trials', 7 August 1998.

Chapter 3

1   Poupard JA and Miller LA. (1992). Biological warfare. In *Encyclopedia of Microbiology*, Volume 1 (pp. 297-308). New York: Academic Press.

2   Goldblat J. (1971). *The Problem of Chemical and Biological Warfare Volume IV: CB Disarmament Negotiations 1920-1970.* Stockholm: Almqvist and Wiksell.

3   Jelsma J. (1995). Military implications of biotechnology. In M Fransman *et al.* (Eds.), *The Biotechnology Revolution* (pp. 284-97). Oxford: Blackwell.

4   Dando MR. (1994). *Biological Warfare in the 21st Century: Biotechnology and the Proliferation of Biological Weapons.* London: Brassey's.

5   Perry Robinson J. (1996). Some lessons for the Biological Weapons Convention from preparations to implement the Chemical Weapons Convention. In O Thränert (Ed.), *Enhancing the Biological Weapons Convention* (pp. 86-113). Bonn: Dietz.

6   Sims NA. (1988). *The Diplomacy of Biological Disarmament: Vicissitudes of a Treaty in Force, 1975-85.* London: Macmillan.

7   Smith JE. (1996). *Biotechnology* (3rd Edition). Cambridge (for the Institute of Biology): Cambridge University Press.

8   Office of Technology Assessment. (1991). *Biotechnology in a Global Economy.* OTA-BA-494. Washington DC: US Congress.

9   Lelieveld HLM. (1996). Safe biotechnology. 7. Classification of microorganisms on the basis of hazard. *App. Microbiol. Biotechnol.*, 45, 723-9.

10   Pearson GS. (1998). The threat of deliberate disease in the 21st century. In AE. Smithson (Ed.), *Biological Weapons Proliferation: Reasons for Concern, Courses of Action.* Washington DC: The Henry L. Stimson Center.

11   Russian Federation. (1992). *Illustrative List of Potential BW Agents.* BWC/CONF.III/VEREX/WP.23, 7 April. Geneva: United Nations.

12   Russian Federation. (1992). *Illustrative List of Potential BW Agents.* BWC/CONF.III/VEREX/WP.23, 7 April. Geneva: United Nations.

13   Depositary States. (1980). New Scientific and Technological Developments to the Convention on the Prohibition of the Development, Production and Stockpiling of Bacteriological (Biological) and Toxin Weapons and on Their Destruction. In *Report of the Preparatory Committee for the Review Conference of the Parties to the*

Convention on the Prohibition of the Development, Production and Stockpiling of Bacteriological (Biological) and Toxin Weapons and on Their Destruction. BWC/CONF.1/5, 6 February. Geneva: United Nations.

14   United Nations. (1980). *Text of the Final Declaration of the First Review Conference.* BWC/CONF.I/10. Appendix III. In J Goldblat and T Bernauer (1991) *The Third Review of the Biological Weapons Convention: Issues and Proposals.* UNIDIR Research Paper No. 9. New York:United Nations.

15   Armstrong FB *et al.* (1981). *Recombinant DNA and the Biological Warfare Threat.* DPG-5450A, May. US Army Test and Evaluation Command, Dugway Proving Ground.

16   International Center for Defense Analysis. (1985). *Implications of Present Knowledge and Past Experience for a Possible Future Chemical/Conventional Conflict (II).* NTIS, AD- A153656, January. Alexandria, Virginia. Prepared for the Office of the Undersecretary of Defense for Research and Engineering.

17   United Nations. (1986). Text of the Final Declaration of the Second Review Conference. BWC/CONF.II/13/II. Appendix IV. In J Goldblat and T Bernauer (1991) *The Third Review of the Biological Weapons Convention: Issues and Proposals.* UNIDIR Research Paper No. 9. New York: United Nations.

18   Hunger I. (1996). Article V: Confidence Building Measures. In GS Pearson and MR Dando (Eds.), *Strengthening the Biological Weapons Convention: Key Points for the Fourth Review Conference* (pp 77-92). Geneva: QUNO.

19   Dando MR. (1994). *Biological Warfare in the 21st Century: Biotechnology and the Proliferation of Biological Weapons.* London: Brassey's.

20   Dando MR. (1996). New developments in biotechnology and their impact on biological warfare. In O Thränert (Ed.), *Enhancing the Biological Weapons Convention* (pp. 21- 56). Bonn: Dietz.

21   Dando MR. (1996). Article I: Scope. In GS. Pearson and MR. Dando (Eds.), *Strengthening the Biological Weapons Convention: Key Points for the Fourth Review Conference* (pp. 7-30). Geneva: QUNO.

22   Dando MR and Pearson GS. (1997). The Fourth Review Conference of the Biological and Toxin Weapons Convention: Issues, outcomes, and unfinished business. *Politics and the Life Sciences,* 16 (1), 105-26.

23   Jaurin B *et al.* (1987). *Genetic Engineering and Biological Weapons.* Umea, Sweden: FOA Report A 40058-4.4, National Defense Research Institute. (Translated from the Swedish by the Office of International Affairs, National Technical Information Service, Springfield, VA, USA in May 1988).

24   Dubuis B. (1994). *Recombinant DNA and Biological Warfare.* Swiss Federal Institute of Technology, Zurich: Institute for Military Security Technology (IMS).

25   United Kingdom. (1991). In United Nations *Background Document on New Scientific and Technological Developments Relevant to the Convention on the Prohibition of the Development, Production and Stockpiling of Bacteriological (Biological) and Toxin Weapons and on Their Destruction.* BWC/CONF.III/4, 26 August (pp. 18-26). Geneva: United Nations.

26   United Nations. (1991). *Final Declaration of the Third Review Conference of the Parties to the Convention on the Prohibition of the Development, Production and Stockpiling of Bacteriological (Biological) and Toxin Weapons and on Their Destruction.* BWC/CONF.III/23, 9-27 September. Geneva:United Nations.

27   Dando MR and Pearson GS. (1997). The Fourth Review Conference of the Biological and Toxin Weapons Convention: Issues, outcomes, and unfinished business. *Politics and the Life Sciences* 16:105-26.

28   Canada. (1991). *Novel Toxins and Bioregulators: The Emerging Scientific and Technological Issues Relating to Verification and the Biological and Toxin Weapons Convention.* Ottawa, September.

29   United States. (1996). In United Nations *Background Paper on New Scientific and Technological Developments Relevant to the Convention on the Prohibition of the Development, Production and Stockpiling of Bacteriological (Biological) and Toxin Weapons and on Their Destruction.* BWC/CONF.IV/4, 30 October (pp. 18-26). Geneva:United Nations.

30   United Nations. (1996). *Final Declaration of the Fourth Review Conference of the Parties to the Convention on the Prohibition of the Development, Production and Stockpiling of Bacteriological (Biological) and Toxin Weapons and on Their Destruction.* BWC/CONF.IV/9, 25 November- 6 December. Geneva: United Nations.

31   Montecucco C and Papine E. (1995). Cell penetration of bacterial protein toxins. *Trends in Microbiology*, 3, 165-8.

32   Dando MR.(1996). New developments in biotechnology and their impact on biological warfare. In O Thränert (Ed.), *Enhancing the Biological Weapons Convention* (pp. 2-56). Bonn: Dietz..

33   Weatherall D. (1995). *Science and the Quiet Art: Medical Research and Patient Care.* Oxford: Oxford University Press.

34   United Kingdom. (1996). In United Nations *Background Paper on New Scientific and Technological Developments Relevant to the Convention on the Prohibition of the Development, Production and Stockpiling of Bacteriological (Biological) and Toxin Weapons and on Their Destruction.* BWC/CONF.IV/4, 30 October (pp. 7-18). Geneva:United Nations.

35   United Nations. (1996).*Final Declaration of the Fourth Review Conference of the Parties to the Convention on the Prohibition of the Development, Production and Stockpiling of Bacteriological (Biological) and Toxin Weapons and on Their Destruction.* BWC/CONF.IV/9, 25 November-6 December. Geneva: United Nations.

36   Pearson GS. (1990). The CBW spectrum. *The ASA Newsletter*, 90, 1 and 7-8.

37   Pearson GS. (1990). The CBW spectrum. *The ASA Newsletter*, 90, 1 and 7-8.

38   Bovallius A. (1997). NBC in the 21st century. *The ASA Newsletter*, 97, 1 and 3-4.

39   Sawyer D. (1998). *Germ Warfare: Weapons of Terror.* Script of *Prime Time*, ABC News, (pp. 1-38), 25 February.

40   Alibeck K. (1998). Russia's deadly expertise. *New York Times*, 27 March.

41 Preston R. (1998). Annals of warfare: The bioweaponeers. *The New Yorker*, March, pp. 52-65.

42 Geissler E. (1995). *The BW Activity Zigzag*. Paper presented to the Pugwash Meeting No. 212, 2-3 December, Geneva.

43 Weiner T. (1998). Defector details Soviet germ project. *International Herald Tribune*, 26 February.

44 Yankulin Y. (1997). Plague syndrome or the purgatory of one of the creators of bacteriological warfare. *Moscow Izvestya*, 15 October, pp. 5. (FBIS translated text).

45 Akimov P. (1988). The military aspect of developing bioengineering. *Zarubezhnoye voyennoye obozreniye*, 8, 16-20. (*Soviet Press Selected Translations*, Nov/Dec, 1989).

46 Alibeck K. (1998). Russia's deadly expertise. *New York Times*, 27 March.

47 Preston R. (1998). Annals of warfare: The bioweaponeers. *The New Yorker*, March, 52-65.

48 Alibeck K. (1998). Russia's deadly expertise. *New York Times*, 27 March.

49 Alibeck K. (1998). Russia's deadly expertise. *New York Times*, 27 March.

50 Preston R. (1998). Annals of warfare: The bioweaponeers. *The New Yorker*, March, 52-65.

51 Preston R. (1998). Annals of warfare: The bioweaponeers. *The New Yorker* March, 52-65.

52 Pearson GS. (1998). The threat of deliberate disease in the 21st century. In A E Smithson (Ed.), *Biological Weapons Proliferation: Reasons for Concern, Courses of Action*. Washington DC: The Henry L. Stimson Center.

53 Sandakjchiev LS. (1997). *Directions of R & D Restructuring of State Research Centre of Virology and Biotechnology "VECTOR"*. Paper presented to a NATO Advanced Research Workshop on 'Conversion of Former BW Facilities — a Chance for the Development and Production of Prophylactic, Diagnostic and Therapeutic Measures for Countering Diseases', 5-9 November, Budapest.

54 Spertzel, RO et al. (1994). *Biological Weapons Proliferation: Technical Report*. DNA-MIPR-90-715, April. US Army Medical Research Institute of Infectious Diseases, Fort Detrick, MD.

55 Rogers P and Dando MR. (1994.) A *Violent Peace: Global Security After the Cold War*. London, Brassey's.

56 Spertzel RO et al. (1994). *Biological Weapons Proliferation: Technical Report*. DNA-MIPR-90-715, April. US Army Medical Research Institute of Infectious Diseases, Fort Detrick, MD.

57 Erlich J. (1997). Pentagon panel warns of smaller chem-bio attacks. *Defense News*, 1-7 December, pp. 12.

58 Starr B. (1998). Experts study chemical threat to Pentagon. *Jane's Defence Weekly*, 18 February, 4.

59 US Army Foreign Science and Technology Center. (1993). *Advances in Chemical Science — Foreign: New Developments in Microencapsulation.* DST-1820S-363-93, July. Washington DC: Defense Intelligence Agency.

60 Graham B. (1997). Fears of germ warfare ignite the Pentagon. *International Herald Tribune,* 17 December, pp. 3.

61 Armstrong FB *et al.* (1981). *Recombinant DNA and the Biological Warfare Threat.* DPG-5450A, May. Dugway Proving Ground: US Army Test and Evaluation Command.

62 United States Army. (1983). *Biological Warfare Threat Study.* USA CMLS Threat Section, 6 October.

63 Dando MR. (1996). New developments in biotechnology and their impact on biological warfare. In O Thränert, (Ed.), *Enhancing the Biological Weapons Convention* (pp. 21-56.) Bonn: Dietz.

64 Almond JW. (1997). Understanding the molecular basis of infectious disease: Implications for biological weapons development. In R. Ringer (Ed.), *The Devil's Brews I: Chemical and Biological Weapons and Their Delivery Systems.* Babrigg Memorandum 16, Centre for Defence and International Studies, Lancaster University.

65 Potter CW. (1987). Influenza. In A. J. Zuckerman *et al.* (eds), *Principles and Practice of Clinical Virology* (pp. 199-225). Chichester: John Wiley.

66 Cohen W. (1997). *Proliferation: Threat and Response.* Washington DC: Department of Defense (Text from WorldWideWebsite http://www.defense link.mil/pubs/prolif 97/index.html).

67 Cohen W. (1997). *Proliferation: Threat and Response.* Washington DC: Department of Defense. (Text from WorldWideWebsite http://www.defense link.mil/pubs/prolif 97/index.html).

68 United States Army. (1983). *Biological Warfare Threat Study.* USA CMLS Threat Section, 6 October.

69 Devine KM. (1995). The *Bacillus subtilis* genome project: Aims and progress. *Tibtech,* 13, 210-16.

70 Hoch JA. (1993). Regulation of phosphorelay and initiation of sporulation in *Bacillus subtilis. Ann. Rev. Microbiol.,* 47, 441-65.

71 Setlow P. (1995). Mechanisms for the prevention of damage to DNA in spores of *Bacillus* species. *Ann. Rev. Microbiol.,* 49, 29-54.

72 Starr B. (1997). DARPA begins research to counter biological pathogens. *Jane's Defence Weekly,* 15 October, 8.

73 Miller J and Broad WJ. (1998). Secret exercise finds US can't cope with a biological terror attack. *International Herald Tribune,* 27 April, pp. 3.

74 Cohen W. (1997). *Proliferation: Threat and Response.* Washington DC: Department of Defense. (Text from WorldWideWebsite http://www.defense link.mil/pubs/prolif 97/index.html).

75 Weatherall D. (1995). *Science and the Quiet Art: Medical Research and Patient Care.* Oxford: Oxford University Press.

76 Turney J. (1998). Probing the great divide. *The Times Higher Education Supplement,* 27 February, pp. 23.

Chapter 4

1   Larres K. (1998). Aliens knocking at the door. *The Times Higher Education Supplement,* 20 March, p 29.

2   Fein H. (1990). Genocide: A sociological perspective. *Current Sociology,* 38, 1-7.

3   Osmańczyk EJ. (1990). Genocide Convention. In *The Encyclopedia of the United Nations and International Relations* (pp. 328-9). London: Taylor and Francis.

4   Osmańczyk EJ. (1990). Genocide Convention. In *The Encyclopedia of the United Nations and International Relations* (pp. 328-9). London: Taylor and Francis.

5   Deen T. (1998). Annan slams UN failure to prevent ethnic wars. *Jane's Defence Weekly,* 18 February, 4.

6   United Kingdom. (1996). New Scientific and Technological Developments Relevant to the Biological and Toxin Weapons Convention. In United Nations, *Background Paper on New Scientific and Technological Developments Relevant to the Convention on the Prohibition of the Development, Production and Stockpiling of Bacteriological (Biological) and Toxin Weapons and on Their Destruction.* (pp. 7-18). BWC/CONF.IV/4, 30 October. Geneva: United Nations.

7   Creasy Col WM. (1950). *Presentation to the Secretary of Defense's Ad Hoc Committee on CEBAR,* 24 February. Declassified 29 August 1977.

8   Smith JR. (1997). Playing hide-and-seek with Iraq's warheads. *International Herald Tribune,* 22-3 November, pp. 2.

9   Raineri V. (1980). Germ war lab in Oakland ? Does the Navy have a germ warfare lab? *People's World,* 19 April, pp. 1 and 4.

10 Conadera A. (1981). Cultured killers: Biological weapons and Third World targets. *Science for the People,* July/August, 16-20.

11 Ottaway DB. (1988). US links Soviets to disinformation. *Washington Post,* 17 January, pp. A3.

12 United Kingdom. (1996). New Scientific and Technological Developments Relevant to the Biological and Toxin Weapons Convention. In United Nations, *Background Paper on New Scientific and Technological Developments Relevant to the Convention on the Prohibition of the Development, Production and Stockpiling of Bacteriological (Biological) and Toxin Weapons and on Their Destruction.* (pp. 7-18). BWC/CONF.IV/4, 30 October. Geneva: United Nations.

13 Starr B. (1997). Cohen warns of new terrors beyond CW. *Jane's Defence Weekly,* 4 June, 27.

14   Starr B and Evers S. (1997). Interview: US Secretary of Defense, William Cohen. *Jane's Defence Weekly*, 13 August, 32.

15   Anon. (1983). 'Ethnic weapons': Apartheid's final solution? In *Resister: Bulletin of the Committee on South African War Resistance. No. 23: Chemical Warfare Threat* (pp. 13-17). London: January.

16   Mohan CR. (1984). Ethnic weapons? *Strategic Analysis*, VII , 555-9.

17   Thatcher G. (1988). Genetic weapon: Is it on the horizon? *Christian Science Monitor*, 15 December, B11-12.

18   Larson CA. (1970). Ethnic weapons. *Military Review*, November, 3-11.

19   Anon. (1992). Race weapon is possible. *Defense News*, 7, 23 March, pp. 2.

20   Bartfai T *et al.* (1993). Benefits and threats of developments in biotechnology and genetic engineering. In Appendix 7A of *SIPRI Yearbook 1993*, Pp 293-305. Oxford: Oxford University Press, (for the Stockholm International Peace Research Institute).

21   Human Genome Organization. (1998). *Human Genome Project: Frequently Asked Questions.* Update of 20 April on Website (http://hugo.gdb.org/).

22   Schuler GD *et al.* (1996). A gene map of the human genome. *Science*, 274, 25 October, 540-5.

23   Pennisi E. (1998). A Planned Boost for Genome Sequencing, But the Plan is in Flux. *Science*, 281, 10th July, 148-149.

24   Lander ES. (1996). The new genomics: Global views of biology. *Science*, 274, 25 October, 536-9.

25   Tjian R. (1995). Molecular machines that control genes. *Scientific American*, February, 38-45.

26   Lander ES. (1996). The new genomics: Global views of biology. *Science*, 274, 25 October, 536-9.

27   Kuper A. (1994). *The Chosen Primate: Human Nature and Cultural Diversity.* Cambridge, MA: Harvard University Press.

28   Marks J. (1995). *Human Biodiversity: Genes, Race, and History.* New York: Aldine de Gruyer.

29   Cummings MR. (1994). *Human Heredity: Principles and Issues.* St. Paul: West Publishing Company.

30   Mourant AE. (1983). *Blood Relations: Blood Groups and Anthropology.* Oxford: Oxford University Press.

31   Marks J. (1995). *Human Biodiversity: Genes, Race, and History.* New York: Aldine de Gruyer.

32   Cummings MR. (1994). *Human Heredity: Principles and Issues.* St. Paul: West Publishing Company.

33   Cummings MR. (1994). *Human Heredity: Principles and Issues.* St. Paul: West Publishing Company.

34   Ruvolo M. (1997). Genetic diversity in hominoid primates. *Ann. Rev. Anthropol, 26*, 515-40.

35   Marks J. (1995). *Human Biodiversity: Genes, Race, and History*. New York: Aldine de Gruyer.

36   Marks J. (1995). *Human Biodiversity: Genes, Race, and History*. New York: Aldine de Gruyer.

37   Ruvolo M. (1997). Genetic diversity in hominoid primates. *Ann. Rev. Anthropol, 26*, 515-40.

38   Martin PD. (1997). DNA: The invisible evidence. *Biologist, 44*, 306-9.

39   Shriver MD *et al.* (1997). Ethnic-affiliation estimation by use of population-specific DNA markers. *Am. J. Hum. Genet, 60*, 957-64.

40   Committee on DNA Forensic Science. (1996). *The Evaluation of Forensic DNA Evidence: An Update*. Washington, D.C: National Academy Press.

41   Sweden. (1996). Background Information on New Scientific and Technological Developments Relevant to the Biological and Toxin Weapons Convention. In *Background Paper on New Scientific and Technological Developments Relevant to the Convention on the Prohibition of the Development, Production and Stockpiling of Bacteriological (Biological) and Toxin Weapons and on Their Destruction* (pp. 2-7). BWC/CONF.IV/4/Add.1., 21 November. Geneva: United Nations.

42   Zhang W-W *et al.* (1995). Advances in cancer gene therapy. *Advances in Pharmacology, 32*, 289-341.

43   Wagner JA. and Gardner P. (1997). Toward cystic fibrosis gene therapy. *Ann. Rev. Med, 48*, 203-16.

44   Anderson WF. (1998). Human Gene Therapy. *Nature;* 392, 30th April, Supp 25-29.

45   Friedman T. (1997). Overcoming the obstacles to gene therapy. In *Special Report: Making Gene Therapy Work* (pp. 96-101) Scientific American, June, 95-123.

46   Culver KW. (1994). *Gene Therapy: A Handbook for Physicians*. Des Moines: Mary Ann Liebert.

47   United Kingdom. (1996). New Scientific and Technological Developments Relevant to the Biological and Toxin Weapons Convention. In United Nations, *Background Paper on New Scientific and Technological Developments Relevant to the Convention on the Prohibition of the Development, Production and Stockpiling of Bacteriological (Biological) and Toxin Weapons and on Their Destruction*. (pp. 7-18). BWC/CONF.IV/4, 30 October. Geneva: United Nations.

Chapter 5

1   Franck RE Jr and Hildebrandt GG. (1996). Competitive aspects of the contemporary military-technical revolution: Potential military rivals to the US. *Defense Analysis*, 12, 239-58.

2   Starr B. (1997). Countering weapons of mass destruction. *Jane's Defence Weekly*, 12 November, 39-40.

3   Goldman FG. (1997). *The International Legal Ramifications of United States Counter-Proliferation Strategy*. The Newport Papers No. 11, United States Naval War College.

4   Thomas E *et al.* (1997). Saddam's dark threat. *Newsweek*, 24 November, pp. 10-17.

5   DeSutter P. (1997). Deterring Iranian NBC use. *Strategic Forum*, No. 110, April. Institute for National Strategic Studies, National Defense University, Washington DC.

6   Opall B. (1996). Study: N. Korea can win by waging bio-chem war. *Defense News*, 11, 4-10 November, pp. 3 and 18.

7   Drozdiak W. (1997). Albright urges NATO to fight arms of mass destruction. *International Herald Tribune*, 17 December, pp. 1 and 10.

8   Roberts B. and Pearson GS. (1998). Bursting the biological bubble: How prepared are we for biowar? *Jane's International Defense Review*, 4, 21-4.

9   Zanders JP. (1997). *Chemical Weapons Between Disarmament and Non-Proliferation*. Stockholm: SIPRI.

10 Moore M. (1996). World Court says mostly no to nuclear weapons. *Bulletin of the Atomic Scientists*, September/October, 39-42.

11 Brodie I. (1997). Iraq faced threat of nuclear attack. *The Times*, 22 December, pp. 2.

12 Erlich J. (1998). New US nuclear policy maintains ambiguity. *Defense News*, 5-11 January, pp. 4 and 19.

13 Brodie I. (1997). Iraq faced threat of nuclear attack. *The Times*, 22 December, pp. 2.

14 Erlich J. (1998). New US nuclear policy maintains ambiguity. *Defense News*, 5-11 January, pp. 4 and 19.

15 Utgoff VA. (1997). *Nuclear Weapons and the Deterrence of Biological and Chemical Warfare*. Occasional Paper No. 36, October. Henry L. Stimson Center, Washington DC.

16 Doty P. (1997). *Surviving in the Long Term*. Paper presented at the 47th Pugwash Conference on Science and World Affairs, 1-7 August, Lillehammer.

17 Meselson M and Perry Robinson JP. (1995). *Outline for an Integrated Approach to the Problem of Biological Weapons*. Paper presented to Pugwash Meeting No. 212, 2-3 December, Geneva.

18 Moodie M. (1995). Beyond proliferation: The challenge of technology diffusion. *The Washington Quarterly*, 18, 183-202.

19 Bailey KC. (1995). Responding to the threat of biological weapons. *Security Dialogue*, 26, 383-97

20   Collins JM et al. (1994). *Nuclear, Biological and Chemical Weapon Proliferation: Potential Military Countermeasures.* Report for Congress, July. Congressional Research Service, Washington DC.

21   Dando MR. (1998). The development of international legal constraints on biological warfare in the 20th century. *Finnish Yearbook of International Law.* In press.

22   Nadelmann EA. (1990). Global prohibition regimes: The evolution of norms in international society. *International Organization, 44,* 479-526.

23   Tanzman EA. (1995). *Arms Control and the Rule of Law.* Paper presented to the 36th Annual Convention of the International Studies Association, February, Chicago.

24   Tanzman EA. (1995). *Arms Control and the Rule of Law.* Paper presented to the 36th Annual Convention of the International Studies Association, February, Chicago.

25   Croft S. (1996). *Strategies of Arms Control: A History and Typology.* Manchester: University Press.

26   Tanzman EA. (1995). *Arms Control and the Rule of Law.* Paper presented to the 36th Annual Convention of the International Studies Association, February, Chicago.

27   Leonard, Ambassador JF. (1997). Keynote Address: The control of biological weapons: Retrospect and prospect. In J Tucker (Ed.), *Inspection Procedures for Compliance Monitoring of the Biological Weapons Convention.* CGSR-97-002, December. Monterey Institute of International Studies and Center for Global Security Research, Lawrence Livermore National Laboratory.

28   United Nations. (1993). *Report: Ad Hoc Group of Government Experts to Identify and Examine Potential Verification Measures from a Scientific and Technical Standpoint.* BWC/CONF.III/VEREX/9, September. Geneva: United Nations.

29   United Nations. (1994). *Final report: Special Conference of the States Parties to the Convention on the Prohibition of the Development, Production and Stockpiling of Bacteriological (Biological) and Toxin Weapons and on Their Destruction.* BWC/SPCONF/1, October. Geneva: United Nations.

30   United Nations. (1994). *Final report: Special Conference of the States Parties to the Convention on the Prohibition of the Development, Production and Stockpiling of Bacteriological (Biological) and Toxin Weapons and on Their Destruction.* BWC/SPCONF/1, October. Geneva: United Nations.

31   Pearson GS. (1996). Article VI: Lodging of complaints with and their investigation by the Security Council. In G S Pearson and M R Dando (Eds.), *Strengthening the Biological Weapons Convention: Key Points for the Fourth Review Conference,* (pp. 93-7). Geneva: QUNO.

32   United Nations. (1997). *Procedural Report of the Ad Hoc Group of the States Parties to the Convention on the Prohibition of the Development, Production and Stockpiling of Bacteriological (Biological) and Toxin Weapons and on Their Destruction.* Eighth Session, BWC/AD HOC GROUP/38, 6 October. Geneva: United Nations.

33   University of Bradford/Stockholm International Peace Research Institute. (1998). Joint CBW Project Website (http://www.brad.ac.uk/acad/sbtwc).

34   Tóth, T. (1997). A window of opportunity for the BWC Ad Hoc Group. *The CBW Conventions Bulletin*, 37, 1-5.

35   Dando MR. (1998). *Implications of a Strengthened Biological and Toxin Weapons Convention for the Biotechnology and Pharmaceutical Industry*. Paper presented to a European Federation of Biotechnology meeting on 'A Strengthened Biological and Toxin Weapons Convention: Potential Implications for Biotechnology'. 28-9 May, Vienna.

36   Dando MR. (1998). The development of international legal constraints on biological warfare in the 20th century. *Finnish Yearbook of International Law*. In press.

37   Dando MR. (1997). Strengthening the Biological Weapons Convention: Moving towards the endgame. *Disarmament Diplomacy*, 21, 10-14.

38   Colombia. (1998). *Statement by the Non-Aligned Movement and Other Countries*, March. Mission Permanente de Colombia, Geneva.

39   Office of the Press Secretary. (1998). *Fact Sheet: The Biological Weapons Convention*, 27 January. The White House, Washington DC.

40   European Union. (1998). *Common Position: Relating to Progress Towards a Legally Binding Protocol to Strengthen Compliance with the Biologial and Toxin Weapons Convention (BTWC) and the Intensification of the Work in the Ad Hoc Group to that End*, 25 February. European Union, Brussels.

41   Steinberg JB. (1997). *Address by the Deputy Assistant to the President for National Security Affairs*, 9 June. Carnegie Endowment for International Peace, Washington DC.

42   Pearson GS. (1998). An action plan for the Ad Hoc Group of the Biological and Toxin Weapons Convention. *The ASA Newsletter*, 98, pp. 1 and 12-13.

43   Lebeda FJ. (1997). Deterrence of biological and chemical warfare: A review of policy options. *Military Medicine*, 162, 156-61.

44   Buchanan Captain HL. (1997). Poor man's A-bomb? *Proceedings of the US Naval War College*, April, 83-6.

45   Thränert O. (1997). Biological weapons and the problem of proliferation. *Aussenpolitik*, 11, 148-57.

46   Pearson GS. (1993). Prospects for chemical and biological arms control: The web of deterrence. *The Washington Quarterly*, Spring, 145-62.

47   Pearson GS. (1993). Prospects for chemical and biological arms control: The web of deterrence. *The Washington Quarterly*, Spring, 145-62.

48   Wheelis M. (1997). *Addressing the Full Range of Biological Warfare in a BWC Compliance Protocol*. Paper presented to Pugwash Meeting No. 229, 20-21 September, Geneva.

49   Wheelis M. (1997). *Addressing the Full Range of Biological Warfare in a BWC Compliance Protocol*. Paper presented to Pugwash Meeting No. 229, 20-21 September, Geneva.

50   Wheelis M. (1997). *Addressing the Full Range of Biological Warfare in a BWC Compliance Protocol.* Paper presented to Pugwash Meeting No. 229, 20-21 September, Geneva.

51   United Nations. (1998). *Report of the United Nations Special Commissions Team to the Technical Evaluation Meeting on the Proscribed Biological Warfare Programme.* (Vienna, 20- 27 March). New York: United Nations.

52   Deen T. (1997). Cuba accuses USA of 'biological aggression'. *Jane's Defence Weekly,* 14 May, 8.

53   Wright S. (1997). Bioweapons: Cuba case tests treaty. *Bulletin of the Atomic Scientists,* November-December, 18-19.

54   Working Group on Biological Weapons Verification. (1996). *Report of the Subgroup on Investigations of Alleged Use or Release of Biological or Toxin Weapons Agents,* April. Federation of American Scientists, Washington D.C.

55   Tucker JB. (1998). Strengthening the BWC: Moving toward a compliance protocol. *Arms Control Today,* January/February, 20-7.

56   United Kingdom. (1974). *Biological Weapons Act 1974.* London: HMSO.

57   Sims NA. (1996). Article IV: National implementation. In GS Pearson and MR Dando (Eds.), *Strengthening the Biological Weapons Convention: Key Points for the Fourth Review Conference* (pp. 45-58). Geneva: QUNO.

58   Zilinskas RA. (1990). Terrorism and biological weapons: Inevitable alliance? *Perspectives in Biology and Medicine,* 34, 44-72.

59   Deutch J. (1997). Terrorism. *Foreign Policy,* Fall, 10-22.

60   Vegar J. (1998). Terrorism's new breed. *Bulletin of the Atomic Scientists,* March/April, 50-5.

61   Norqvist A. and Sandstrom G. (1997). *How Prepared is the Civilian Society for Biological Weapon Attack?* Paper presented to Pugwash Meeting No. 229, 20-21 September, Geneva.

62   Starr B. (1996). Chemical and biological terrorism. *Jane's Defence Weekly,* 14 August, 16-21.

63   Cohen WS. (1997). Preparing ourselves to combat terror weapons. *International Herald Tribune,* 27 November, p 5.

64   Ferguson JR. (1997). Biological weapons and US law. *Journal of the American Medical Association,* 278, 357-60.

65   Perry Robinson J. (1992). Chemical and biological weapons proliferation and control. In *Proliferation and Export Controls: An Analysis of Sensitive Technologies and Countries of Concern.* London: Saferworld.

66   Tucker JB. (1998). Strengthening the BWC: Moving toward a compliance protocol. *Arms Control Today,* January/February, 20-7.

67   Subrahmanyam K. (1993). Export controls and the North-South controversy. *The Washington Quarterly,* Spring, 135-43.

68   Tucker JB. (1998). Strengthening the BWC: Moving toward a compliance protocol. *Arms Control Today*, January/February, 20-7.

69   Tóth, T. (1997). A window of opportunity for the BWC Ad Hoc Group. *The CBW Conventions Bulletin*, 37, 1-5.

70   Huxsoll DL. (1995). The US Biological Defense Research Programme. In B Roberts (Ed.), *Biological Weapons: Weapons of the Future?* Significant Issues Series, XV, 58-67. Center for Strategic and International Studies, Washington D.C.

71   Pearson GS. (1995). Chemical and biological defence: An essential national security requirement. *RUSI Journal*, August, 20-7.

72   Yamamoto KR. (1989). Retargeting research on biological weapons. *Technology Review*, 92, 23-4.

73   Rutman RJ and Disch HJ. (1990). Commentary on articles by Charles F Dasey and Thomas R Dashiell on the Biological Defense Research Program (BDRP). *Politics and the Life Sciences*, 9, 117-21.

74   Beal C. (1995). The invisible enemy. *International Defense Review*, 3, 36-41.

75   Howell Captain R D. (1995). BIDS — What is it? How does it work? *Army Chemical Review*, January, 33-5.

76   Dando MR. (1997). *Technologies for Monitoring the Biological and Toxin Weapons Convention: An Emerging Consensus?* Paper presented to the NATO ARW on 'Monitoring the Environment for Biological Hazards', 19-22 May, Warsaw.

77   Hewish M. (1997). Surviving CBW: Detection and protection. *International Defense Review*, 3, 30-48.

78   Franz D *et al*. (1997). Clinical recognition and management of patients exposed to biological warfare agents. *Journal of the American Medical Association*, 278, 399-411.

79   Crossette B. (1998). UN experts assert Iraq hides germ weapons. *International Herald Tribune*, 10 April, pp. 1 and 12.

80   Leitenberg M. (1996). *The Desirability of International Sanctions Against the Use of BW, Against Violation of the BWC, and Against False Allegations of Use.* Paper presented to the 5th Workshop of the Pugwash Study Group on Implementation of the Chemical and Biological Weapons Convention, 21-22 September, 1996.

Chapter 6

1   Mobley Col JA. (1995). Biological warfare in the twentieth century: Lessons from the past, challenges for the future. *Military Medicine*, 160, 547-53.

2   Pearson GS. (1998). *The Protocol to Strengthen the BTWC: An Integrated Regime.* Paper presented at the CBW Protection Symposium, 10 May, Stockholm.

3   Pearson GS. (1998). *The Protocol to Strengthen the BTWC: An Integrated Regime.* Paper presented at the CBW Protection Symposium, 10 May, Stockholm.

4   Dimond H, Leklem EJ. (1998). Iraq strikes new deal on inspections at special sites. *Arms Control Today*, January/February, 29&35.

5   UNSCOM. (1998). *Report of the United Nations Special Commission's Team to the Technical Evaluation Meeting on the Proscribed Biological Warfare Programme (Vienna, 20-27 March).* 1 April. New York: United Nations.

6   United Nations. (1998). *Report of the Executive Chairman on the Activities of the Special Commission Established by the Secretary-General Pursuant to Paragraph 9 (b) (i) of Resolution 687 (1991).* S/1998/332, 16 April. New York: United Nations.

7   Goshko JM. (1998). UN inspectors in Iraq foresee resistance. *International Herald Tribune*, 16 April, pp. 8.

8   Wright S. (1992). Prospects for biological disarmament. *Transnational Law and Contemporary Problems*, Fall, 453-85.

9   Dando MR. (1997). *Biotechnology in a Peaceful World Economy.* Paper presented to a NATO Advanced Research Workshop on 'Conversion of Former BW Facilities — A Chance for the Development and Production of Prophylactic, Diagnostic and Therapeutic Measures for Countering Diseases', 5-9 November, Budapest.

10   Islam S and von Gierke U. (1998). *Infectious Diseases and Poverty.* Paper presented to the 47th Pugwash Conference on Science and World Affairs, 1-7 August, Lillehammer.

11   Krause RM. (1992). The origin of plagues: Old and new. *Science*, 257, 1073-8.

12   Cohen ML. (1992). Epidemiology of drug resistance: Implications for a post-antimicrobial era. *Science*, 257, 1050-5.

13   Le Guenno B. (1995). Emerging viruses. *Scientific American*, October, 30-7.

14   Berkelman RL *et al.* (1994). Infectious disease surveillance: A crumbling foundation. *Science*, 264, 368-70.

15   Plotkin BJ and Kumball AM. (1998). Designing an international policy and legal framework for the control of emerging infectious diseases: First steps. *Emerging Infectious Diseases*, January-March, 1-11.

16   Zilinskas RA. (1992). Confronting biological threats to international security: A biological hazards early warning program. *Annals New York Academy of Sciences*, 666, 147-76.

17   Wheelis ML. (1992). Strengthening biological weapons control through global epidemiological surveillance. *Politics and the Life Sciences*, 11, 179-89.

18   Woodall J. (1996). *ProMED-mail: Reporting Unusual Outbreaks through the Internet.* Paper presented to Pugwash Meeting No. 219, 21-22 September, Geneva.

19   Meeting Report. (1996). Programme for countering emerging infectious diseases (ProCEID) by prophylactic, diagnostic and therapeutic measures. *Biologicals*, 24, 71-4.

20   Cole LA. (1996). The Specter of Biological Weapons. *Scientific American*, 275, 60-65.

21   Kaplan DE and Marshall A. (1996). 'The Cult at the End of the World! The Incredible Story of Aum'. London: Hutchinson.

22   Cole LA. (1996). The Specter of Biological Weapons. Scientific American, 275, 60-65.

23   Roberts B and Moodie M. (1998). Combating NBC Terrorism: An Agenda for Enhancing International Cooperation. Washington, D.C: Chemical and Biological Arms Control Institute.

24   Preston R. (1998). Discuss biological weapons. International Herald Tribune, 22 April, pp. 3.

25   Lowe K et al. (1995). Protective Values of a Simple BW Protective Mask. Alexandria, Virginia and Porton Down, UK: Institute for Defense Analyses, Chemical and Biological Defence Establishment.

26   Roberts B and Moodie M. (1998). Combating NBC Terrorism: An Agenda for Enhancing International Cooperation. Washington, D.C: Chemical and Biological Arms Control Institute.

27   France. (1997). Preliminary Working Document Submitted by France on Behalf of the Group of Seven Major Industrialized Countries and the Russian Federation: International Convention for the Suppression of Terrorist Bombings. A/AC.252/L.2, 11 February. New York: United Nations.

28   Hothelet RC. (1997). A forum for international justice. Christian Science Monitor, 25 August (Editorial).

29   Blitz J. (1998). UN war crimes court agreed. Financial Times, 18/19 July, pp. 2.

30   Coupland RM. (1996). The effects of weapons: Defining superfluous injury and unnecessary suffering. Medicine and Global Survival, 3, 1-6.

31   Meselson M. (1998). Strengthening the BWC and Criminalising Biological Weapons under International Law. Chemical and Biological Conventions Bulletin, December.

32   Meselson M. (1998). Strengthening the BWC and Criminalising Biological Weapons under International Law. Chemical and Biological Conventions Bulletin, December.

33   Ratner SR. (1998). International law: The trials of global norms. Foreign Policy, Spring, 65-80.

34   Keohane RO. (1998). International institutions: Can interdependence work? Foreign Policy, Spring, 83-96.

35   Preston R. (1998). Discuss biological weapons. International Herald Tribune, 22 April, pp. 3.

36   Barnaby W. (1997). The Plague Makers: The Secret World of Biological Warfare. London: Satin Publications.

37   Preston R. (1998). Discuss biological weapons. International Herald Tribune, 22 April, pp. 3.

38   Short N. (1998). A new model for arms control? The strengths and weaknesses of the Ottawa Process and Convention. Disarmament Diplomacy, 24, 7-11.

Chapter 7

1   Kutukdjian GB. (1997). *For a World Commission on the Ethics of Scientific Knowledge and Technology.* Paper presented by the Director of the UNESCO Bioethics Unit to the 47th Pugwash Conference on Science and World Affairs, 1-7 August, Lillehammer.

2   Mobley Col JA. (1995). Biological warfare in the twentieth century: Lessons from the past, challenges for the future. *Military Medicine,* 160, 547-53.

Index